Praise for *The Calorie Myth*

"In *The Calorie Myth*, readers will find that all calories *are not* the same, and that focusing on the *kinds* of foods they are eating, rather than just the quantity of food, can boost their brain power, help them lose the extra ten pounds, and create a life that promotes long-term health. I highly recommend this book."

—Daniel G. Amen, MD, bestselling author of
Change Your Brain, Change Your Body

"*The Calorie Myth* will do more to assist people with their health than all the popular diet books currently out there put together. I want to shout, 'Bravo! Finally someone gets it!' "

—Christiane Northrup, MD, OB/GYN, bestselling author of
Women's Bodies, Women's Wisdom and *The Wisdom of Menopause*

"Jonathan Bailor presents a weight-loss program that is based on rigorous science. Far from 'just another diet book' . . . it can help you turn the tide of weight gain."

—Joann E. Manson, MD, MPH, DRPH, Harvard University

"*The Calorie Myth* provides a clear plan for readers to reset their metabolism and shed excess weight—not through excessive exercise and restrictive calorie counts, but with delicious, nourishing foods and moderate exercise. A valuable and transformative book."

—Mike Moreno, MD, bestselling author of *The 17 Day Diet*

"*The Calorie Myth* is a proven and practical guide to fighting the big problem of obesity. Simplifying a bunch of biology while making decades of academic obesity research accessible to everyone, Bailor gives a complete and captivating explanation of the science of losing weight permanently."

—Dr. Theodoros Kelesidis, Division of Endocrinology, Diabetes, and
Metabolism, Harvard Medical School, UCLA School of Medicine

"Brilliant. *The Calorie Myth* is a masterful compilation of nutritional and exercise science disproving the archaic fat-loss theory of 'eat less, exercise more.' Bailor persuasively packages a wealth of research along with his personal and professional experience into an easily understood and applied framework that will change the way you live, look, and feel. For all those who feel left behind in the nutritional battles and exercise gimmicks of the last ten years, look no further. Bailor will end your confusion once and for all."

—Dr. William Davis, *New York Times* bestselling author of *Wheat Belly*

"In *The Calorie Myth*, Bailor demolishes the dietary and nutritional nonsense that has contributed to the epidemics of obesity and diabetes in our country. In its place he erects a simple program anyone can follow that is based on solid science and common sense. *The Calorie Myth* is likely to be the last diet book you will ever need to buy. Unless you enjoy failed diets, do the right thing—the healthy thing—and read this book."

—Dr. Larry Dossey, *New York Times* bestselling author of *Reinventing Medicine*

"When it comes to the most important part of your life, your health, Bailor has written a book that is a must-read for knowing the truth about evaporating body fat. I am a firm believer in achieving the body you have always dreamed of, and Bailor opens the black box of fat loss and makes it simple for you to explore the facts. Read this book today in order to live your best life."

—Joel Harper, *Dr. Oz Show* fitness expert; celebrity personal trainer at joelharperfitness.com

"*The Calorie Myth* reveals some of the latest and best scientific research on the real story of diet, exercise, and their effects on us. Bailor's concept of high-quality exercise is rapidly gaining support in the medical community and has repeatedly delivered clinical results which seem almost too good to be true. I heartily recommend this book to people who want to take responsibility for their own health."

—Dr. John J. Ratey, Clinical Professor of Psychiatry, Harvard Medical School; author of *Spark: The Revolutionary New Science of Exercise and the Brain*

"*The Calorie Myth* sheds light on the surprising discrepancy between the way healthy nutrition has been presented to the public and the science that underlies it. The idea that fat in the diet translates into fat on the body has dominated nutritional discussions for decades. This work challenges this central idea, and offers clues about why diabetes has been on the rise, and why so many people who are intent on losing weight have found it so difficult to do so. It is an important work."

—Dr. Anthony Accurso, Johns Hopkins Bayview Medical Center

"As someone who takes fitness and health seriously and has written extensively on this topic over some thirty years, I am generally underwhelmed whenever I see a new how-to book enter the marketplace. *The Calorie Myth* represents something different. Strikingly different in fact. Jonathan Bailor has that rare gift of being able to take highly technical scientific data and interpret them in a way that the average person can understand instantly. But most important, he is able to take that mountain of scientific data and divine the practical and simple direction it is pointing to in terms of advancing human health and fitness. The book you are holding in your hands can be said to represent the thinking person's guide to exercise and diet in the twenty-first century. No fads. No gimmicks."

—John Little, author of *Max Contraction Training*;
coauthor of *Body by Science*

"Revolutionary. Thoroughly researched, rigorously simplified, and downright fun, Bailor's work stands head and shoulders above the mass of fat-loss myths lining bookstore shelves. In his surprising and scientifically sound exposé of the modern fat-loss mythology, Bailor reveals the sources of our fat-loss struggles and provides straightforward, practical solutions. Everyone, and I mean everyone, will learn and laugh a lot while reading *The Calorie Myth*."

—Dr. Jan Fridén, Distinguished Professor,
University of Gothenburg, Sweden

"WOW! This book will blow your mind and is a must-read for anyone who wants to learn how to be healthy the twenty-first-century way. In *The Calorie Myth*, Bailor exposes the dietary myths of why we as a nation are still overweight despite years of bestselling diet books. Calories, fat, exercise, and hormones—it is all in this book and finally someone got it right. The diabesity epidemic stops here."

—Dr. Fred Pescatore, bestselling author of *The Hamptons Diet*

"*The Calorie Myth* redefines and updates the science of weight loss and bravely takes on long-held beliefs about body change. This book provides a groundbreaking paradigm shift for all of those who have struggled with weight loss. I have used this science in my clinic for years. It gets results and changes lives."

—Jade Teta, ND, CSCS; author of *The New ME Diet*

"In *The Calorie Myth*, Bailor entertains as much as he educates. Simplifying and integrating an amazing amount of important scientific and clinical research, Bailor presents a well-conceived, well-researched, and well-written book, in addition to a very sensible, practical, and successful approach to losing fat. This book will undoubtedly change the way you think and look, while keeping you smiling all along the way."

—Dr. Wayne Westcott, Director of Quincy College Fitness Research;
author of *Get Stronger, Feel Younger*

"*The Calorie Myth* is the go-to source for all that is practical, realistic, and effective when it comes to weight loss. Bailor brilliantly brings together all the outdated myths (eat less, exercise more) and dispels them one at a time in a fun, easy-to-understand way. This book changes the future of permanent weight loss forever!"

—Cynthia Pasquella, CHLC, CWC; board certified clinical nutritionist

"This is not just another diet book. Bailor has assembled a wealth of scientific evidence showing how our 'healthy' diet and exercise obsession are making us fat and sick. *The Calorie Myth* is a scientifically backed, paradigm-shifting, and entertaining exposé that disproves our basic ideas of eating and exercise. If you buy one health book this decade, make it *The Calorie Myth*."

—Marion G. Volk, MHSc; obesity researcher

"*The Calorie Myth* is both fun and informative. It challenges the central dogma of diet and weight control and provides a sensible alternative to the current 'less food, more exercise' strategy. Bailor provides a compelling, simple, and practical solution to the challenge of obesity."

—Dr. Steve Yeaman, Deputy Director of
the Institute of Cellular Medicine, Newcastle University

"Jonathan Bailor does an excellent job of explaining why losing weight and achieving a healthy lifestyle are not all about counting calories. His simple approach lends itself well to a broad range of readers, from those just getting started in their education about how foods nourish us (or don't) to those who are well versed in nutrition and healthy living, and who will find his book to be a valuable must-have addition to their library."

—Nell Stephenson, author of *Paleoista* and
coauthor of *The Paleo Diet Cookbook*

THE
CALORIE
MYTH

THE
CALORIE
MYTH

How to Eat More, Exercise Less, Lose Weight, and Live Better

JONATHAN BAILOR

HARPER WAVE

An Imprint of HarperCollins*Publishers*

This book is written as a source of information only. The information contained in this book should by no means be considered a substitute for the advice of a qualified medical professional, who should always be consulted before beginning any new diet, exercise, or other health program. All efforts have been made to ensure the accuracy of the information contained in this book as of the date published. The author and the publisher expressly disclaim responsibility for any adverse effects arising from the use or application of the information contained herein.

HarperCollins books may be purchased for educational, business, or sales promotional use. For information, please e-mail the Special Markets Department at SPsales@harpercollins.com.

A hardcover edition of this book was published in 2014 by HarperWave, an imprint of HarperCollinsPublishers.

FIRST HARPERWAVE PAPERBACK EDITION PUBLISHED 2015.

Previously published in a different form as *The Smarter Science of Slim* by Aavia Publishing in 2012.

Designed by Ruth Lee-Mui
Workout illustrations designed by Alex McVey

Author photo by Bala Sivakumar

Library of Congress Cataloging-in-Publication Data has been applied for.

ISBN: 978-0-06-226734-4 (pbk.)

15   16   17   18   19   OV/RRD   10   9   8   7   6   5   4   3   2   1

To my best friend, partner, and wife, Angela. Just the thought of you brings me more joy, more satisfaction, and more life than anything else I have ever experienced. You are my beloved, without reservation or qualification, as we dance into eternity.

To my heroes and parents, Mary Rose and Robert. All that I am is thanks to your love, example, and support. From the day I was born, and every day after, you have always found a way to help and love me. I live, hoping to return the favor.

Contents

Foreword

Had "official" agencies and other sources of conventional dietary advice gotten the nutrition and health message right to begin with, there would be no need to have so many books on the topic. But they got it wrong—*colossally* wrong.

Ever since the U.S. Department of Agriculture and the U.S. Department of Health and Human Services issued the first U.S. Dietary Guidelines for Americans in 1980, the dietary and health-care communities all synchronized their message for nutrition and health: cut total and saturated fat, eat more "healthy whole grains," watch calories, and increase physical activity.

They advised us that the human body is a vessel that behaves according to the physical laws of thermodynamics: the human body transacts energy currency just like any other energy-consuming vessel—no differently, say, from an automobile or furnace. We are thereby subject to physical laws such as "Calories in, calories out," regardless of whether those calories are in the form of carbohydrate, fat, or protein. According to this line of thinking, it does not matter what hormonal or metabolic environment a calorie enters; the end result is the same.

We were also told that weight gain was a simple matter of consuming more calories than we burned. We were advised that weight loss would occur, predictably and mathematically, when we cut calories *in* or burned more calories *out*, the basis for the "Eat less, exercise more" mantra for maintaining healthy weight. By this line of logic, cutting back, for instance, on the 238 calories in 2 tablespoons of extra-virgin olive oil in your salad while maintaining an unchanged level of physical activity should predictably yield weight loss of 1 pound every two weeks, or 25 pounds over a year. Alternatively, performing housework, such as vacuuming and sweeping the house 30 minutes per day, without altering calorie intake should burn in the neighborhood of 110 calories, yielding just under 12 pounds lost over one year. Easy, eh?

As the nationwide experience has demonstrated, this doesn't work. While there are surely people who are indeed gluttonous and lazy and could be illustrative examples of the "calories in, calories out" concept, there are plenty of people who have followed conventional advice to reduce fat, consume more whole grains, etc., yet now hold an extra 30, 50, 150 pounds on their frame. If there has been a miscalculation, it has been a miscalculation of epic proportions. Could the one in three Americans now obese and another one in three overweight all be gluttonous and lazy? Or is there something fundamentally wrong with the concept of calories in, calories out?

The year 1980 marks this astounding turn of events for the American public: the start of an unprecedented and dramatic increase in calorie intake, weight gain, and overweight and obesity. We now have the worst epidemic of obesity and all the diseases that accompany it, such as hypertension, diabetes, "high cholesterol," degenerating joints, and other conditions, in human history. There surely have been periods in our history when widespread illness plagued us, but those periods were due to mass starvation, war, and disease. In contrast, we have our modern epidemic during a period of virtually limitless abundance.

It doesn't take an astute student of modern culture to see that conventional wisdom is not just inaccurate, but devastatingly wrong. Of course, the human body follows the laws of physics and energy, but not by the simplistic rules offered by conventional dietary thinking.

Anyone who has had some false starts and stops in weight loss learns some tough lessons acquired through the school of hard knocks. For one, cutting calories makes you hungry and miserable, while—though you are not conscious of this—reducing your level of physical activity. Conversely, increasing physical activity creates hunger and increases calorie intake. The combination of the two—decreasing calorie intake while purposefully increasing physical activity—is an especially unpleasant experience and an effort that requires monumental willpower to follow, as it generates ravenous, intense hunger. This last painful strategy, by the way, typically results in dramatic reductions in metabolic rate and loss of muscle mass, both of which further boobytrap any genuine effort at fat loss.

In *The Calorie Myth*, Jonathan Bailor presents the wealth of science we *already* have that (1) should cause us to reject the miserably incorrect "calories in, calories out" misconception; and (2) shows us how to use the very same science to understand the *real* ways the body responds to calories and physical activity. He educates readers on why the human body protects its set-point as a fail-safe survival mechanism, explaining that the only effective, long-term weight-maintenance strategy is to manage your set-point—not to eat less and exercise more.

What is magical about *The Calorie Myth* is the easy-to-grasp, step-by-step way he tells the story, taking the reader by the hand and showing us why this one nutritional insight was misinterpreted and led to catastrophically misguided dietary advice, and how new insights can be keys to unlocking hidden wisdom. He creates a new language and framework that allow readers to put their arms around these concepts without getting bogged down in science, detail, or dogma. Knowledge is power, and in this instance, the proper understanding of just how the human body transacts energy empowers the reader to regain control over metabolism, health, and weight, even after a lifetime of being led astray.

But there is much more here than an unemotional recounting of the nutritional science that makes the case against the myth that "a calorie is a calorie is a calorie." Jonathan captures the essence of effective nutritional arguments in his own clear, succinct, and uniquely clever way. The same no-holds-barred, incisive thinking goes into Jonathan's analysis of exercise, educating the reader on why "less is more" once the principles of hormonal correction and high-intensity bursts of exercise are understood using the revolutionary insight of *eccentric* exercise.

This book is appropriately titled: it does indeed bash the myths underlying how the human body manages energy. There is no hypothesizing or empty prediction here; there is detailed analysis of the science underlying these principles—principles that, when properly and consistently applied, achieve heights of functioning, result in weight loss, and provide relief from the myriad health conditions of modern life.

—William Davis, MD, author of the number one *New York Times* bestseller *Wheat Belly: Lose the Wheat, Lose the Weight, and Find Your Path Back to Health* and *The Wheat Belly Cookbook*

Preface

The dual epidemics of obesity and type 2 diabetes are the looming public health crises of the twenty-first century. All around us today, in all walks of life, are people who struggle with weight control. The growing prevalence of obesity in the United States and around the world, especially among children and adolescents, portends an enormous global burden of chronic disease in the future. The crystal ball shows not only more people with diabetes, but also enormous numbers of people with hypertension, heart disease, stroke, and even cancer. Although medical research has made strides in treating and controlling some of the health consequences of obesity, the prevention and management of obesity truly hold the key to improved health. Of particular importance, we now know that people suffering from overweight or obesity can take charge of their health—if they are willing to make even modest changes in their lifestyle.

Throughout my career in preventive medicine and epidemiology, I, together with my colleagues, have valued the importance of empowering the public through information and shared decision making. Our research has focused on prevention of cardiovascular disease and diabetes, including assessing the role of lifestyle factors in reducing risks. We have examined the "power of prevention" in several large-scale clinical studies, including the Harvard Nurses' Health Study, the Women's Health Initiative, the Women's Health Study, the VITamin D and OmegA-3 TriaL (VITAL), and other research projects. One of the major findings from our large population-based studies is that type 2 diabetes and heart disease are largely preventable through lifestyle modifications, which are powerful determinants of our risk of chronic disease. For example, we've published papers from the Nurses' Health Study indicating that at least 90 percent of cases of type 2 diabetes and at least 80 percent of heart attacks can be prevented by lifestyle changes, including being physically active, maintaining a healthy weight, and following a diet that is high in fruits, vegetables, and whole grains and low in saturated and trans fats and refined carbohydrates.

We've made efforts to inform the public of these findings, as well as of the work of other researchers around the world, often writing columns in magazines and working closely with print and electronic media over the years. Yet the scientific findings of so many researchers and other dedicated individuals in academia remain largely unknown by the general public. Part of the problem is the pervasive and over-powering impact of mass marketing by the food industry. Another problem is the often confusing and contradictory messages about nutri-tion and health on the Internet and various mass media outlets. Even the dietary guidelines from the federal government may seem confusing and at odds with some of the research studies that have attracted at-tention. How is the general public supposed to know which scientific studies to believe?

That's why Jonathan Bailor has performed an invaluable service with his book *The Calorie Myth*. Jonathan has studied thousands and thousands of pages of academic research on health and weight loss and he has put the results into terms that the ordinary person can under-stand. We have made great strides over the years in understanding how the body responds to different types of food. Yet all too often a popular author cites the scientific evidence selectively, emphasizing only those aspects of the wide-ranging research that support the diet plan he or she is promoting. Jonathan's work is far from "just another diet book."

The Calorie Myth dismantles the myths that have contributed enor-mously to the health and weight problems that many people have and replaces them with easy-to-understand facts that will change the way you think about eating and exercise. On the eating side, he shows why changes in a person's metabolism affect weight gain and how to get your metabolism burning rather than storing body fat. He pro-vides a sensible formula for eating the right kinds of food that produce satiety—that fill you up so much that you won't have room for the types of foods that are fueling the obesity and diabetes epidemics. He shows how balance is the key to long-term health and weight loss. He also clarifies what the scientific literature suggests are the best ways to exercise. Short bursts of vigorous and forceful activity can provide all the stimulation needed to get your metabolism back on track. But moderate exercise also has a role.

The scientific community now knows a great deal about how the human body works. In culling the literature and gathering the results of so many clinical studies, Jonathan Bailor presents a weight-loss program that is based on rigorous science. We can make the right choices that will help us to avoid becoming overweight or obese. As a treasure trove of reliable information and sound facts, *The Calorie Myth* can help you take charge of your destiny and turn the tide on weight gain.

—JoAnn E. Manson, MD, MPH, DrPH, Professor of Medicine and the Michael and Lee Bell Professor of Women's Health, Harvard Medical School; Chief, Division of Preventive Medicine, Brigham and Women's Hospital

Introduction:
The SANE Solution

In other fields, when bridges do not stand, when aircraft do not
fly, when machines do not work, when treatments do not cure,
despite all conscientious efforts on the part of many persons to
make them do so, one begins to question the basic assumptions,
principles, theories, and hypotheses that guide one's efforts.

—Arthur Jensen, University of California[1]

Over the past few decades, we've been trying harder and harder to
be healthy and fit. The result: we got heavy and sick. What's going on
here? When did healthy and fit start making us heavy and sick? And
why is everyone calling us lazy gluttons?

If a doctor prescribes us a medication and it makes us worse, is
that our fault? No. However, it is up to us to stop taking it and to find a
new doctor. Similarly, if an architect builds us a house and it crumbles,
is that our fault? No. But we'd better find a good contractor who knows
how to build something solid and safe.

We have to apply the same logic to health and fitness. We've re-
ceived so much contradictory, damaging advice over the years—often
resulting in frustration and extra pounds. It's high time for us to make a
better choice. But what other option do we have than the decades-old
calorie-counting approach?

I have good news and bad news. Scientific and technological advancements have been just as amazing in the health, fitness, and fat-loss arenas

over the past forty years as they have been everywhere else. But here's the bad news: nobody's told us about them. The field of modern nutrition and exercise science has provided a proven alternative, and it does not involve complex calorie counting, confusing workout routines, or other gimmicks.

We can think about the modern approach to avoiding obesity and diabetes as we would the modern approach to avoiding lung cancer: No need to track breaths in and breaths out—just enjoy clean air. Don't avoid everything. Just steer clear of things proven to poison your lungs. Similarly, no need to track calories in and calories out—just enjoy so much delicious healthful (what I call "SANE") food that you are too full for the ("inSANE") foods that poison your body.

We've gotten worse while trying harder because we've been written a bad prescription and given a faulty blueprint. The traditional approach to health and fitness is like attempting to avoid lung cancer by smoking *light* cigarettes and jogging. We're still destroying our respiratory system—albeit more slowly—and even some well-intentioned jogging cannot undo that damage.

Likewise, eating less of a traditional diet and doing more traditional exercise does not prevent obesity and diabetes. It may delay them, but the diet still destroys our metabolic system—albeit more slowly—and the exercise does not undo that damage. Fortunately, we have the solution: we can use simple and proven science to make "healthy" healthy again.

WE CAN LIVE BETTER

Starting in the 1970s, diet and nutrition experts reduced food and exercise down to a lowest common denominator: calories. They told us that we just need to eat fewer calories and exercise more to burn them off. It doesn't matter what we eat. "There are no bad foods," they said, "only bad quantities. *Everything* in moderation." In this same spirit, many experts claimed the type of exercise we do is irrelevant—as long as we get our heart rate up for a certain amount of time so that we burn a lot of calories.

This dual set of recommendations led to a world where nearly half of all women and a third of all men are following a diet plan while the fitness industry has blossomed into a $30 billion business that employs more than half a million people. In other words, we trusted the experts and took the calorie-counting concept to heart. Here is what that has done to our hearts (and waistlines):

US HEALTH AND WEIGHT TRENDS

Millions of Nonfatal Heart Disease Incidents

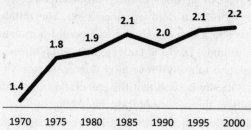

1970	1975	1980	1985	1990	1995	2000
1.4	1.8	1.9	2.1	2.0	2.1	2.2

Millions of Hospital Discharges for Cardiovascular Diseases

1970	1975	1980	1985	1990	1995	2000	2006
3.3	4.4	5.1	5.5	5.2	5.8	6.3	6.2

Percent of Americans at Least Overweight

'71-'74	'76-'80	'88-'94	'99-'02	'03-'04	'07-'08
40%	40%	57%	65%	66%	68%

Millions of Americans with Diabetes

'71-'74	'76-'80	'88-'94	'99-'02	'03-'04	'07-'08
4.5	5.6	8.1	13.6	15.2	18.8

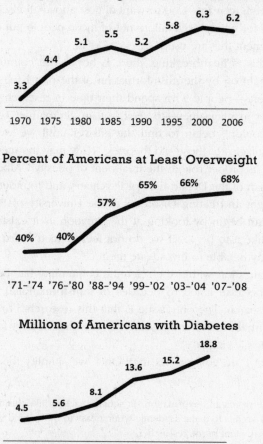

Judging by these results, the calorie-counting approach is not effective. We're trying, but it's not working—anywhere. The worldwide rate of obesity has more than doubled since 1980. The number of people who are overweight today equals the total world population a century ago. Most disturbingly, David S. Ludwig, MD, PhD, director of the New Balance Foundation Obesity Prevention Center, Boston Children's Hospital, reports, "Obesity is such that this generation of children could be the first basically in the history of the United States to live less healthful and shorter lives than their parents."[2] In the words of Susan Wooley, cofounder of the Eating Disorder Clinic at the University of Cincinnati College of Medicine: "The failure of [overweight]* people to achieve a goal they seem to want—and to want almost above all else—must now be admitted for what it is: a failure not of those people but of the methods of treatment that are used."[3]

While this is heartbreaking, there is hope. The counterproductive results brought on by the misinformation of the past have led contemporary experts—people who spend their time in research labs, not on television or in magazines—to seek out an alternative. These experts knew we couldn't begin to find the answer until we were ready to admit the fallacies of those old theories. "How may the medical profession regain its proper role in the treatment of obesity?" Albert Stunkard, MD, chairman of the Department of Psychiatry and founder of the Center for Weight and Eating Disorders at the University of Pennsylvania, asks. "We can begin by looking at the situation as it exists and not as we would like it to be. . . . If we do not feel obliged to excuse our failures, we may be able to investigate them."[4]

This realization within the scientific community has been wonderful for us because it led to decades of transformational fat loss and wellness research. The only issue is that this research, buried in dense medical journal articles and research papers, has not yet found its way out of academic circles.

You and I are going to fix that. Once we simplify this science, we

---

* You will see words and explanations in square brackets [like this] in quotes from researchers. I do this to make academic writing easy to understand while maintaining the original intent of the researcher.

can escape the myths at the heart of the obesity, diabetes, and heart disease epidemics. We will experience something truly liberating: we will see how accurate information makes it easy to get slim and be healthy.

Does that sound too good to be true? Have you ever met anyone who eats as much as he or she wants, does not exercise, and still stays skinny? We all have. So the question is not: "Is simple lifelong slimness possible?" Millions of naturally thin people have already demonstrated that it is. The question is: "How can I burn fat automatically, like naturally thin people?"

Along the same lines, have you ever met anyone who easily avoids foods most of us crave? Again, we all have. The question is not: "Is it possible to avoid foods that many people crave?" Millions of vegetarians demonstrate every day that it's possible to resist drive-thru burgers for life. The question is: "How can we get our minds to see harmful foods in the way that vegetarians' minds see meat?"

The modern science of health and fitness has revealed a surprising and encouraging answer: We don't need to eat less and exercise more—harder. We can eat more and exercise less—*smarter*.

Smarter is the key. The focus should be on food and exercise quality instead of quantity. By eating plenty of higher-quality food and doing less (but higher-quality) exercise, we unconsciously avoid overeating and provide our body with a unique combination of nutrition and hormones, one that reprograms the body to behave more like one of a naturally thin person. Likewise, psychologists have pioneered techniques we can use to reprogram the way our mind perceives food. If we dedicate a few hours to freeing our mind, it can free us from the cravings that sabotage our efforts.

We're virtually dying to know the facts about fat loss and health, but who has time to examine thousands of pages of scientific studies? It took me over a decade of being sleep deprived, sending countless e-mails, and calling researchers around the world to understand twelve hundred nutrition and exercise studies and integrate them into this book. Thankfully, you won't need a decade to absorb this information—you just need a few hours to read it and five weeks to allow it to change your life.

I've simplified my findings into a five-week plan and free online program (www.SANESolution.com) to burn fat and shed pounds quickly, and a flexible lifestyle program that improves your health and helps you slim down permanently. You'll learn:

- How supposedly "healthy" foods cripple our ability to burn fat
- How to burn fat while eating more food
- How to get all the benefits of exercise in a tenth of the time
- How eating less sets us up to gain fat in the long run
- How a few minutes of a new form of exercise immunize us against fat gain
- How we fix the underlying hormonal condition causing us to gain fat

To start, let's look at a point-by-point comparison of the 1970s calorie-counting theory and the 2010s smarter science of slim. On the left you will find the advice you've read dozens of times. Now look at the right-hand column. There is quite a difference.

OUTDATED THEORY VERSUS MODERN SCIENCE

The Calorie Myth Eat Less, Exercise More—Harder	The SANE Solution Eat More, Exercise Less—*Smarter*
Focuses on calorie quantity and ignores calorie quality	Leverages calorie quality to take care of calorie quantity
Fights against our "set-point weight"	Lowers our "set-point weight"
Focuses on short-term weight loss	Focuses on long-term fat loss and health
Slows down our metabolism	Speeds up our metabolism
Ignores hormonal issues	Focuses on hormonal issues
Ensures a profit motive for the diet and fitness industry	Keeps it all simple right from the start so you can heal your body and bank account

To be clear, the "eat less, exercise more" approach can work—just not very often, easily, or enjoyably. Studies show that counting calories does not keep off body fat over the long term, 95.4 percent of the time. To put that into perspective, quitting smoking cold turkey has a 94.5 percent failure rate. Put these two facts together: we are more likely to give up the third most addictive substance in the world (trailing only heroin and cocaine) without any help than we are to shed weight using the "gold-standard" advice you have been taught your whole life (the gospel that I was taught back in my personal trainer days).

The modern, smarter approach is not about better versus worse; it's about simple versus complex: When we're hungry, we eat smarter foods until we're full. When we work out, we do smarter exercise for a shorter period of time.

That's it. Freed from hunger or complicated calculations about how much we're eating or exercising, we can spend our energy on our dreams, jobs, and families. The calorie-counting model is so complex that there are reality TV shows about it, with contestants constantly doing food math and spending life-draining hours in the gym. Worried about how much we're eating or exercising, we have little time or energy for anything else.

Both approaches can get you to "the other side." But while counting calories is like frantically zigzagging through a minefield, eating more and exercising less—but smarter—is as natural and low key as strolling through a meadow.

Consider a study done at Skidmore College comparing a traditional calorie-counting "eat less, exercise more—harder" program against a simpler "eat more, exercise less—smarter" program. Let's call the groups in the study the Harder Group and the Smarter Group.

The Harder Group ate a more conventional Western diet while doing traditional aerobic exercise for forty minutes per day, six days per week. The Smarter Group ate a smarter diet while exercising only 60 percent as much, but with higher quality. The study lasted for twelve weeks and included thirty-four women and twenty-nine men between the ages of twenty and sixty.

At the end of the study, the Harder Group ate less food and exercised eighteen hours more than the Smarter Group. The Smarter Group focused on high-intensity cardio and resistance training, and ate more but higher-quality calories. Here's what the researchers found:

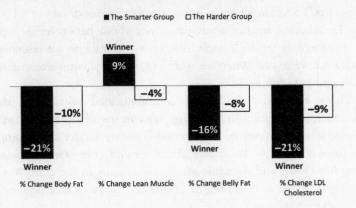

SMARTER VERSUS HARDER

■ The Smarter Group   □ The Harder Group

Intrigued? It gets better. The program in this book takes the strategies used by the Smarter Group to the next level.

We don't use the same surgical techniques we used forty years ago. We don't use the same computers we used forty years ago. And there's no need to use the same nutritional and exercise approaches we used forty years ago. Thousands of studies show a simpler, safer, and more sustainable way to trim off those unwanted pounds while improving every aspect of our health. It is time to free ourselves from outdated Calorie Myths. It is time to enjoy a SANE Solution.

THE CALORIE MYTHS

In the first part of this book, we'll cover the new science that lays the foundation for the program. It may be tempting to skip this section and jump straight into the "how-to" information, but I would caution against that. Without this foundational information, the practical steps later in the book won't make sense because you won't have any context for understanding them. So please give the science a shot. We've given the Calorie Myths decades to confuse us. Let's give the SANE Solution a few short hours to clear things up.

We'll start by digging into research concerning the set-point—a range of about ten pounds that our body works to keep us within. We'll see that processed food creates a hormonal "clog" that raises our set-point weight and causes chronic fat gain. We will also see how healing our hormones and lowering our set-point weight, via high-quality whole plant and animal foods, keeps us slim as reliably as our existing set-point keeps us heavy. We will free ourselves from trying to manually regulate calories in and calories out—a maddening, never-ending task that's just about as feasible as trying to manually regulate all your breaths in and breaths out.

Next, we'll see how the message "A calorie is a calorie, so eat whatever, just not too much" is about as accurate as saying, "Liquid is liquid, so drink whatever, just not too much." We will find that the quality of calories varies wildly and is determined by four factors: Satiety, Aggression, Nutrition, and Efficiency.

Satiety is how quickly calories fill us up.

Aggression is how likely calories are to be stored as body fat.

Nutrition is how many vitamins, minerals, essential amino acids, essential fatty acids, etc., calories provide.

Efficiency is how easily calories are converted into body fat.

Whether a calorie is high quality or low quality depends on where it fits on the SANEity spectrum. High-quality calories are on the healthy end of the SANEity spectrum. They are nonstarchy vegetables, nutrient-dense proteins, whole-food fats, and low-fructose fruits. They are Satisfying, unAggressive, Nutritious, and inEfficient. These SANE foods fill us up quickly and keep us full for a long time. SANE foods provide a lot of nutrients and few of them can be converted into body fat. Even better, SANE foods trigger the release of body-fat-burning hormones, clear clogs, and lower our set-point. The more SANE foods we eat, the simpler slim becomes.

Low-quality calories are just the opposite. Starches and sweets are on the unhealthy end of the SANEity spectrum. They are unSatisfying, Aggressive, nonNutritious, and Efficient. When we eat these inSANE foods we have to overeat to satisfy ourselves. These inSANE foods provide few nutrients and they are easily converted into body fat. Triggering the release of body-fat-storing hormones, inSANE foods cause clogs and raise our set-point. The more inSANE foods we eat, the more complex slim becomes.

Next, you and I will walk through research revealing why the quality of our calories is so important. We will discover how calorie quality controls the hormones that control our set-point. We'll also see how the clogged-up and myth-filled food world of today has a long history. One of the lowest-quality sources of calories in the world is starch, but our government refuses to recognize this fact. In its pyramid and plate, starches are promoted vigorously as though they should be the cornerstone of a healthy diet. We'll see how big food, fitness, and pharmaceutical corporations exploit these government guidelines and graphics to keep people and profits fat.

THE SOLUTIONS: GET SANE AND SMART

Here's where we'll get practical. You and I will cover how to put the science we learned into practice in our everyday lives to achieve long-term fat loss and health. We will see that SANE eating is enjoyable and sustainable. When we eat an abundance of high-quality whole food, our tastes will change, our cravings will disappear, and we will be too full to be tempted with processed low-quality food. Eating more SANE food causes the quality of our diet to rise. This rise lowers our set-point, and our body begins to work more like the body of a naturally thin person.

We'll also explore the wide disconnect between what we've been taught about exercise and what researchers have proved. We'll explore how exercising to enable our body to burn fat for us long term is completely different from exercising to burn a few calories right now. We will see how moving our body slowly, safely, and forcefully speeds the metabolic healing at the heart of making slim simple. We will see how, far from making us bulky, smarter resistance training is the key to staying slim and healthy. We'll then wrap up by exploring how to exercise smarter.

THE FIVE-WEEK SANE SOLUTION PLAN

In the last part of the book, I will offer you a complete five-week mental, nutritional, and physical plan that will forever free you from yo-yo dieting and optimize your health. You will get access to exclusive apps, interactive online programs, at-home exercise videos, recipes, meal plans, and much more at www.SANESolution.com. We'll work through mental activities that enable us to overcome subconscious roadblocks that could impede our fat-loss efforts regardless of how much science we know. We'll discover psychological tools that enable us to easily eliminate the desire for inSANE foods. We'll see exactly how many servings of SANE foods we need to eat to heal our metabolism and how easy it is to grocery shop, cook, and eat out SANEly. I'll arm you with more than thirty recipes, snacks, and substitutions that speed hormonal healing. Finally, we'll see safe, smarter exercises that we can do at home or at a gym in just twenty minutes per week. (That's not per day—that's per *week*.)

This SANE Solution has dramatically and permanently improved the lives of many people and it will do the same for you. Let's get the myths and misinformation out of the way and make slim simple again. Let's eat smarter, exercise smarter, and live better.

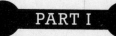

PART I

THE
CALORIE MYTHS

Hippocrates [the father of Western medicine] wrote that the obese should "eat only once a day and . . . walk naked as long as possible." Progress in [the fat-loss] area will require that we move beyond this 2,000-year-old prescription and instead develop strategies that are based on twenty-first-century science.

—Jeffrey M. Friedman, Rockefeller University[5]

The Myth of Calorie Math

The first of the three Calorie Myths at the heart of our fat-loss and health struggles is that calorie counting is required to avoid obesity and disease.

Calorie Myth #1: Weight Loss = Calories In – Calories Out

But reducing the human body to a simple mathematical equation doesn't work. Just as a healthy body automatically balances blood pressure and blood sugar within a normal range, a healthy body also automatically balances the intake and expenditure of calories within a normal range. However, when the body's healthy balance mechanism is broken by low-quality foods, these otherwise unconscious functions become conscious and complex. We manage blood pressure with prescriptions. We regulate blood sugar with insulin injections. We track how many calories we eat and how many steps we take each day. We try to decipher food labels.

We continue to get heavier and sicker while trying harder because the weight-loss prescription we've been written is wrong. The problem is not a lack of calorie counting, pill popping, or insulin injections. Everyone was healthier and slimmer before anyone heard of those things. The problem is that something is breaking our biology and that we're trying to starve, stress, and medicate to address its consequences, instead of fixing the biological breakdown itself.

COMPLEXITY COMES FROM MISINFORMATION

In June 2011, Barry Popkin and Kiyah Duffey, doctors at the University of North Carolina at Chapel Hill, made a startling discovery. They discovered that the number of calories consumed per person per day increased by a jaw-dropping 570 calories between 1977 and 2006. At first glance, it appeared that they definitively demonstrated what many assumed to be the cause of our obesity, diabetes, and heart disease epidemics: we are eating too much.

However, a second glance at their data reveals an even more startling discovery. If the average person is consuming 570 more calories than necessary per day and if the calorie-counting math we hear about daily is accurate, then the average person should have gained 476 pounds since 2006.*

Is it possible that instead of asking, "Why are we getting fatter?" we should be asking, "Why don't all of us weigh six hundred plus pounds?" What could possibly explain the huge disconnect between the quantity of calories we're eating and the quantity of fat we're gaining?

Here are three possible explanations:

1. We're eating less.
2. We're exercising more.
3. The Calorie Math doesn't add up.

Let's start with the first possible explanation: Did we avoid gaining 476 pounds because we cut calories dramatically after 2006? Obesity and lifestyle-related disease rates have continued their upward climb, so this doesn't seem likely. And if we look at the preceding few decades, this explanation just isn't possible.

---

* 570 calories per person per day times 365 days in a year equals 208,050 calories. Multiply this by 8 years and we end up with 1,664,400 excess calories per person between 2006 and 2014. Divide 1,664,400 by the 3,500 calories in a pound of fat and we get 476 pounds of fat per person.

Since the late 1970s, we have gradually worked our way up to eating an additional 570 calories per person per day. But let's estimate that over those few decades, we each ate a more modest 300 additional calories per day. According to traditional calorie math, the average American should have gained 907 pounds of fat between 1977 and 2006.* It seems that we continue to consume more calories, but whatever prevented those excess calories from causing everyone to gain 907 pounds between 1977 and 2006 also prevented each of us from gaining 476 pounds between 2006 and 2014.

Let's look at the second possible explanation: Did we avoid a 476-pound weight gain because our level of physical activity increased dramatically from 2006 to 2014? This theory holds up only if the average person jogged for over an hour and a half every day for the past eight years. That's enough jogging to cross the entire United States eleven times.

That didn't happen.

This possibility also suffers from the same challenge as the first. The exercise explanation doesn't solve the question of how we avoided the previous 907-pound weight gain because, as we've all heard, we've experienced a *drop* in physical activity that is actually believed to be a major *cause* of the obesity epidemic.

That leaves us with the third possible explanation—that we're better off thinking about weight in terms of biology, not math. We've gained only a tiny fraction of those 476 pounds because our body doesn't work like a calculator.

Researchers at the University of Washington cite the role of a complex control system in the brain that adjusts the calories our body takes in and expends, both immediately and over the long term, to achieve homeostasis and keep our "body energy status"—our weight—stable over time. Similarly to the way the body automatically regulates insulin and blood glucose until that system is overwhelmed and breaks down

* 300 calories times 365 days in a year equals 109,500 extra calories per person per year. Multiply that by 29 years we get 3,175,500 excess calories consumed per person between 1977 and 2006. 3,175,500 extra calories divided by 3,500 calories in a pound of fat equals 907 pounds of fat.

(leading to type 2 diabetes), the body automatically regulates body fat until it is overwhelmed and breaks down (leading to overweight and obesity). Another way to think of it: Much as we exhale more when we inhale more, or we urinate more when we drink more, we also burn more when we eat more and burn less when we eat less—automatically. Breaths in and breaths out, water in and water out, and calories in and calories out are matters of established human biology, not mythical metabolic math.

This "burn more when we eat more" behavior explains how we've gained dramatically less than what would be predicted by calorie math. The "burn less when we eat less" behavior explains why studies show traditional calorie-counting approaches failing 95.4 percent of the time—and often provoking even greater rebound weight gain. When we put these two biologic behaviors together, we can see why every weight-loss study ever conducted shows that when people are given a surplus or shortage of calories, they never gain or lose the mathematically anticipated amount of fat. The body just doesn't work that way.

The math myth doesn't work because it assumes our body doesn't do anything to counterbalance our efforts to count calories. The fact is that our genes, brain, and hormones work together to maintain balance, or—as we were taught in our high school biology classes—homeostasis. When it comes to weight, a *healthy* body automatically "counts calories" to maintain a level of fat that is neither too low nor too high.

"The average human consumes one million . . . calories a year, yet weight changes very little," says Jeffrey M. Friedman, MD, PhD, head of the Laboratory of Molecular Genetics at Rockefeller University in New York. "These facts lead to the conclusion that energy balance is regulated with a precision of greater than 99.5 percent, which far exceeds what can be consciously monitored."[6] No one, no matter how meticulous he or she is with a food journal and a calculator, could get that close to perfect.

Losing weight—more specifically, losing fat—and keeping it off seem complex because common calorie-counting approaches fight this system. Traditional "starve your way to success" strategies may make for good television and short-term results, but are sadly ineffective in the long term because we can't win battles against our own biology.

For example, just try to keep yourself from sleeping. Why is keeping yourself from eating any different? Of course we can shave a few hours off our sleep, but that isn't sustainable or healthy. We could also temporarily lose weight by starving ourselves, but that isn't sustainable or healthy either.

As soon as we learn how our body works and how to heal it rather than trying to override it via calorie counting, medication, and spending hours in the gym, we will never have to worry about our weight again. Achieving our health and fitness goals only appears complex because we have been given a whole lot of bad information.

SIMPLICITY THROUGH BIOLOGY

Let's take one last look at how the math myth became ingrained in our culture. I like to compare our lack of progress on the nutrition front to the lack of progress we had on the tobacco front just a few decades ago. Smoking is a good example because it reflects the real world in the early twentieth century—when the public was "educated" about cigarettes by the government and tobacco corporations rather than by the scientific community.

Could you imagine how complex it would be to avoid lung cancer if we were told smoking was harmless?* The modern world of nutrition—where the public is "educated" about eating and exercise by the government and food and fitness corporations rather than by the scientific community—is similar. Just as avoiding lung cancer is much easier once we know the primary cause (smoking), avoiding obesity, diabetes, and heart disease is much easier once we know the cause (eating the wrong foods). However, none of this is possible until someone tells us that cigarette smoke isn't the same as fresh air, and that five hundred calories of nonfat potato chips aren't the same as five hundred calories of spinach and salmon. (It would also be nice if someone ac-

---

* After hearing this analogy one may think, "Fun comparison, but while we can stop smoking, we can't stop eating." This interpretation is a bit off. The scientists aren't telling people to "stop breathing." They identified something that we would be better off not breathing: cigarette smoke. The same thing goes with food. Scientists aren't saying, "Stop eating." They have identified some things that we would be better off not eating: starches and sweets.

knowledged that eating less and exercising more to avoid obesity is like attempting to avoid lung cancer by inhaling less and exhaling more.)

We've automatically avoided 98 percent of the weight we "should" have gained according to calorie counting because our body is designed to balance us out automatically.* It doesn't "want" to be heavy and diabetic any more than it "wants" lung cancer. And just as we can more easily avoid lung cancer by avoiding smoking, we can more easily avoid obesity, diabetes, and heart disease by avoiding low-quality food. When we eat a lot of high-quality food, our set-point takes care of everything else automatically, just as it has successfully done for every other generation that has ever lived.

THE FINAL NAIL IN THE CALORIE-COUNTING COFFIN

In his 2009 article in the journal *Cell Metabolism*, Brent Wisse, MD, of the Diabetes and Obesity Center of Excellence at the University of Washington, noted, "Prior to the discovery of the adipocyte [fat cell] hormone leptin, obesity was thought to result more from a lack of will power than from an underlying biological disorder. Now, 15 years after leptin's discovery, a much different picture of how obesity occurs is beginning to emerge."[7] So, even being conservative, we can say that the calorie-counting approach was considered obsolete by scientists back in 2009. And that's being generous. Actually, way back in 1990, Wayne Miller, PhD, of the Department of Kinesiology at Indiana University, ran a clinical study of the relationship between body fat, energy intake, and exercise and came to the same conclusion: "There was *no* relationship between energy intake and adiposity [body fat]."[8]

The bottom line is that we don't have to worry about regulating life-sustaining bodily functions. That's our brain's and hormones' job. The appetite control center of our brain, the hypothalamus, regulates body weight by precisely balancing the foods we eat, the energy we burn, and the amount of fat on our body. We don't have to "decide" to eat less and exercise more—in fact, says Jeffrey M. Friedman, that simplistic notion is at odds with the substantial scientific evidence that the

---

* The average American gained about twenty pounds during a time period when Americans consumed enough extra calories to gain over thirteen hundred pounds.

set-point is "a precise and powerful biologic system that maintains body weight within a relatively narrow range."[9]

To achieve long-term health and fitness, we need to lower the "relatively narrow range" where Friedman tells us our "precise and powerful biologic system" operates. In order to do that, we need to find out what specifically causes the set-point to rise and how to lower it.

2

Your Set-Point Weight

Think back to high school biology class. We all learned how we pump blood with our circulatory system and how we breathe with our respiratory system. But there is another major system that didn't make it into our high school biology textbooks. This system, at the heart of our weight and health struggles, has been widely ignored by health and fitness experts. It is what scientists call the homeostatic control system, lipostat, adiposity negative feedback system, or more simply, the set-point.

We already understand the idea of the set-point intuitively—we just call it metabolism. We see someone who eats a lot and looks like a beanpole and say, "Sam's so lucky to have a fast metabolism." Or we notice that we're not eating any more or exercising any less but seem to be gaining weight and think, "My metabolism must be slowing down." Little do we know that our intuition is reflecting the last seventy years of biological investigation. What we call a fast metabolism is what researchers call a "low set-point" and what we call a slow metabolism is what researchers call a "high set-point."

Simply put, our set-point is determined by a series of hormonal signals released from our gut, pancreas, and fat cells, which travel to the hypothalamus in the brain. The brain then regulates how much we eat, how many calories we burn, and how much body fat we store long term through various hormones and neurotransmitters, such as serotonin, leptin, and ghrelin.* Our "set-point weight" refers to the level of stored fat our body automatically works to maintain regardless of the quantity of calories we take in or burn off. Our set-point explains why it's so hard to keep fat off through traditional diet and exercise techniques. It also explains why obese people do not keep getting heavier and heavier until they explode.

I know that last part sounds silly, but seriously—why don't obese individuals gain weight forever? If their eating and exercise habits got them to weigh 450 pounds, why won't they eventually weigh 4,500 pounds? These individuals somehow automatically stop gaining weight. How does that work with conventional calorie counting?

It doesn't.

Long-term fat gain works like this: a person's hormones go haywire, causing his set-point weight to rise, and then his body fights to keep him storing more fat. "Obesity is not a disorder of body weight regulation," says David S. Weigle, MD, of the University of Washington School of Medicine and Harborview Medical Center.[10] Most obese people hold a stable weight around their elevated set-point weight. Obesity is simply the result of the body defending this elevated weight—but in a very regulated way. A heavy person's higher set-point prompts the body to store more fat in just the same way that a thin person's lower set-point prompts the body to burn more fat.

We all have a set-point—and *that's* what determines how slim or stocky we are long term. Not calorie counting.

I know this is a huge departure from what we've been told over the past few decades, but look where that information has taken us. Keep in mind that nobody even knew what a calorie was—let alone about counting them—until the concept was introduced to the chemistry community in the mid-1800s. Then it wasn't until the mid-1900s— ironically, just before the beginning of the obesity epidemic—that the

---

* The biological factors involved in our set-point include leptin, insulin, Mc4r receptors, amylin, melanocyte hormones, NPY, peptide YY, galanin, norepinephrine, ART, bombesin, GLP–1, serotonin, urocortin, CRF, agouti-related peptide, ghrelin, mTOR, AMPK, TRH neuron, the thyroid, ARC POMC neuron, Angpt14, gastric inhibitory polypeptide, cholecystokinin, pancreatic polypeptide, and much more. Maybe this is why we haven't heard about it.

concept of calories made it into mainstream diet and health literature. If calorie counting is required for long-term health and fitness, why were the rates of obesity, diabetes, and heart disease so much lower before we even knew what a calorie was?

The explanation is that up until a few decades ago we ate foods that maintained our body's ability to balance calories automatically around a slim set-point weight. In other words, for the past forty years, we've been told to eat things that prevent our body from doing what it did for the entirety of human history—stay healthy and fit, automatically.

To be clear, this isn't controversial. Only two things need to be tested to *prove* that our body works to automatically regulate our body weight around a set-point:

1. If a healthy person eats less of her existing diet, does her body automatically take steps to prevent fat loss? Most simply, does her metabolism slow down?
2. If a healthy person eats more of his existing diet, does his body automatically take steps to prevent fat gain? Most simply, does his metabolism speed up?

Studies have consistently and clearly answered yes to both of these questions. The biochemical *fact* that the body unconsciously regulates body-fat levels within a set range is no more debatable than the fact that the body unconsciously regulates blood sugar within a set range. The days of the set-point "theory" are as long gone as the days of the "theory" that the earth revolves around the sun. We can now overcome obesity by healing—rather than fighting against—the proven biological system that balances our weight.

Do calories count? Of course. But can we really count them—even if we wanted to? As Randy Seely, PhD, director of the Diabetes and Obesity Center at the University of Cincinnati, cleverly tells us: "You couldn't find a scale [sensitive enough to count calories accurately], and if you did, the crumbs you accidentally dropped on the floor would completely throw off your calculations."[11]

Do Calories Count or Not?

Calories count, but that doesn't mean you need to count calories.

—Eric Westman, MD, MHS, Duke University Medical Center

Calories count. However, counting them can't be necessary for health, considering that before most people knew what a calorie was about 90 percent of the population avoided obesity and over 99 percent of us avoided type 2 diabetes.

Think about a sink. If we dump buckets and buckets of water into a sink at once, we're going to have problems. Same thing goes with our body. But nobody pours giant buckets of high-quality calories into his or her body.

Calories count, but why not simplify your life and let your body balance them for you by eating as much as you want, whenever you are hungry, as long as it's high-quality food the body is designed to digest? When you do this, you will drop your set-point, unconsciously consume the appropriate number of calories, take in dramatically more nutrition, overflow with energy, and never feel hungry.

STARTLING SET-POINT STUDIES

In a series of fascinating studies testing the set-point, University of Cincinnati researchers surgically removed and added body fat to various animals. Animals with body fat surgically removed then replaced "exactly the mass of fat which was taken." [12] Animals with body fat surgically added automatically burned more body fat until their body fat returned to its set-point.

In other studies, scientists had human subjects intentionally overeat. The results showed that the participants gained less weight than was predicted by calorie math, stopped gaining weight completely at a certain point, and then eventually returned to their original weight when they stopped overeating. You can see the pivotal role that the set-point plays in our metabolism.

Knowing that our initial set-point is determined by our genetics (studies show 40 percent to 70 percent of weight is genetically determined), researchers also tested twins to prove the power of the set-point. Identical twins share the same genes and therefore the same initial set-point. One study tested two sets: let's call them the Smith twins and the Thomas twins. Given 1,000 excess calories per day, would the Smith twins and Thomas twins all gain the same amount of body fat as predicted by conventional theory, or would the set-point for the Smiths produce a weight gain different from the Thomases'?

Different. Very different.

The Smiths both gained the same amount of weight because they had the same set-point. So did the Thomases. But weight gain varied by nearly four times between the two sets of twins because they had different set-points. For example, while the Smiths each gained two pounds, the Thomas twins each gained eight pounds.

Exercise works the same way. In studies where pairs of twins are put through the same exercise program and have their diets held constant, each pair of identical twins sees the same changes in body composition, but the amount of fat lost varies between the pairs thanks to the varying set-points. Same diets, same exercise, same set-points, same results. Different set-points, different results.

Our set-point determines our long-term weight. If our weight is elevated, it's because our set-point is elevated thanks to what I call a "hormonal clog."

AN ELEVATED SET-POINT IS LIKE A CLOGGED SINK

When our hormones change, our set-point changes. This is why we gain weight as we age. We aren't becoming lazier and hungrier with each passing year (well, maybe a little). As we age our hormones change. The technical term for this is metabolic dysregulation, but it's easier to think of as a hormonal clog.

When we become hormonally clogged, our body can no longer respond to signals from our hormones and brain that otherwise enable us to burn body fat automatically. However, when we increase the quality of our eating and exercise, we can heal our hormones, "unclog," lower our set-point, and get our body to burn fat instead of store fat.

An easy way to understand how this hormonal clog elevates your set-point is to think about your body as being like a sink. When a sink is working properly, more water poured in means more water drains out. The water level may rise temporarily, but the sink will automatically take care of that. The sink is balancing water in and water out at a low level. The sink has a low set-point.

A hormonally healthy body works similarly, doing its best to automatically keep excess fat from sticking around. That's why we each haven't gained the 1,333 pounds we should have gained since the 1970s. A healthy body, like a "healthy" sink, responds to more in with more out, and to less in with less out. Water builds up in sinks, and fat builds up in bodies, only when they become clogged. The key question then is: what causes clogs?

Sinks and bodies become clogged and break down when the wrong *quality* of things are put in them. This is why we don't worry about washing our hands as quickly as possible, but we do work to keep hair out of our drains. We know no *quantity* of the right quality will ever cause our sink to clog. Low quality, not high quantity, causes clogs.

Now, once clogs happen, any amount of water in will cause the water level to rise and stay high. We have a sink with an elevated set-point. What do we do next?

We could use less water for the rest of our lives, or we could use the same amount of water but spend an hour or two per day bailing excess water out of the sink. But why go through all that hassle when we could fix the underlying problem by unclogging the sink and let it balance things out for us automatically around a lower set-point?

Think of our body the same way. When we put the wrong quality of food into it, our body becomes hormonally clogged, causing it to automatically balance us out at an elevated level of body fat. Like a backed-up sink with stagnant water sitting in it, we end up with a bunch of stangnant fat sitting in our body. These clogs can eventually lead to obesity and diabetes.

Once we're clogged and our body is balancing us at an elevated set-point weight, we could eat less of our existing diet, and that would temporarily lower our weight. But why struggle through starvation? That's just like turning the faucet down. It doesn't actually fix anything and it's tough to keep the faucet down forever. We could also do more traditional cardiovascular exercises such as jogging. But why? That's like bailing water out of the sink. It's time consuming and doesn't fix anything long term. The underlying cause of our fat gain persists.

Consider a startling long-term weight-loss study published in the *New England Journal of Medicine*. Fifty men and postmenopausal women forced themselves to eat less for ten weeks and lost weight.[13] Success!

Not so fast. We've all lost weight—the issue is losing it healthfully and keeping it off practically. In response to the study participants' attempts to override their biology, the hormones that regulate their set-points* changed. The result? Their appetite increased and their calorie burn decreased. Biology was trying to return them to their set-point.

Fascinating, but not novel—this finding has been demonstrated in studies for decades. What sets this study apart is what the researchers discovered one year after the starvation diet: many of these alterations in appetite and calorie burn persisted for twelve months after weight loss, even after the start of weight regain. Researchers suggest that the high rate of relapse among obese people who have lost weight has a strong physiological basis and is not simply because they went back to their old habits. Participants who were below their set-point weight still showcased a body engaged in multiple compensatory mechanisms to do everything it could to restore its set-point weight a full year after the calorie-counting "success." Appetite was still increased and "greater-than-predicted" drops in energy expenditure were still observed—the body was "vigorously resisting" the weight loss and trying desperately to regain the weight.[14]

We can avoid this unnecessary hassle and hunger by healing our hormones and restoring our body's ability to balance us out at a lower level of body fat. "If the goal is substantial and sustainable weight loss . . . a more promising approach would be one based upon a strategy of directly altering the set-point. . . . The physiologic adjustments that ordinarily act to resist weight change . . . would instead facilitate the achievement and subsequent maintenance of a lower weight." says Richard Keesey, PhD, of the Department of Psychology at the University of Wisconsin–Madison.[15] By focusing our efforts on restoring the natural set-point, we can stop obsessing over diet and exercise and allow the body to do what comes naturally.

---

* Leptin, ghrelin, peptide YY, cholecystokinin, amylin, gastric inhibitory polypeptide, and more.

Lose 135 Pounds in Twelve Months without
Counting Calories or Being Hungry: Robert's Story

Robert was fed up: "If you think the medical issues that come along with weighing 360 pounds are a challenge, they pale in comparison with the ostracism and low self-confidence that tag along for the ride." Robert had been active and heavy his whole life. He was surrounded by slimmer friends and coworkers who ate more and exercised less than he did.

After countless attempts to get by on 1,200 calories per day, Robert swore off starvation dieting. He could no longer tolerate how terrible it made him feel and the inevitable unhappy ending—after all, he could tolerate being hungry, tired, and depressed for only so long. "Few things are worse than being heavy. Starvation is one of them," Robert says.

When Robert freed himself from the Calorie Myths and embraced the SANE Solution, he immediately felt a sense of hope. "It didn't seem too good to be true because it wasn't saying eat more garbage. But any scientifically backed approach that enables me to eat as much as I want whenever I want, as long as it is 'SANE,' seems doable and sustainable.

"One year after going SANE, I have lost 135 pounds, over a foot around my waist, and I feel better than I did in my twenties. My friends and family can't believe what they are seeing. Heck, I can't believe it either! What makes it work is that I can eat. I don't have to go around counting every calorie; when I am hungry, I eat! If I am hungry 10 times a day, I eat 10 times a day! The difference is I am eating the right stuff."

For the first time in decades, Robert is excited about the future. "I'm not hungry anymore, and the weight is staying off. I've also noticed that even on days when I feel like being naughty, I usually don't feel like going crazy. I can really tell that my set-point is readjusting itself. When you look at a piece of stuffed crust pizza, and go 'Yeah, it looks OK, but, man, all that bread . . . Yuck,' you know something has changed."

3

How Your Set-Point Rises and How to Lower It

I like to think of our set-point weight as being like our set-point body temperature. While the norm might be 98.6°F, your set-point body temperature rises and stays elevated when something is wrong with your body. Both set-point body weight and set-point temperature can be forcibly lowered temporarily via energy deprivation (starvation for body weight and ice baths for body temperature), but since neither of these approaches addresses the root cause, both do more harm than good over the long term.

But when we heal our body, instead of just attending to the symptoms, our body weight and body temperature return to and *stay* at healthy levels. A healthy body automatically maintains a healthy weight in just the same way that it automatically maintains a healthy temperature.

When it comes to this metabolic healing, there are two primary hormones involved with our clog: insulin and leptin. Insulin is produced by the pancreas and through its interaction with our cells and brain, determines whether we are storing or burning fat. Leptin is produced by our body fat and, through its interaction with our gut, central nervous system, and brain, regulates how much food we eat, how much energy we burn, and the amount of body fat specified by our set-point.

Let's assume we are unclogged. When our weight starts rising above our set-point, hormonal signals cause our metabolic rate to go up, our appetite to go down, and our body fat to get burned. This prevents excess fat from sticking around for long. We stay at a slim set-point without trying.

But when we feed our body low-quality foods, it becomes unable to effectively respond to these hormones. Without those hormonal "burn fat" signals, the metabolic processes that otherwise keep us slim do not happen. Once our body is not effectively responding to hormones like leptin and insulin, we become insulin and leptin resistant, and our body starts overproducing these hormones—causing a hormonal clog. For example, some very obese people have been shown to have up to twenty-five times more than a normal level of leptin circulating in their bodies. Chronically high levels of these hormones make our body think that an abnormally high level of body fat is normal. Since our body does its best to balance us at a set-point it thinks is normal, it keeps us at an abnormally high level of body fat. When we eat poorly, we raise our set-point.

A NORMAL SET-POINT

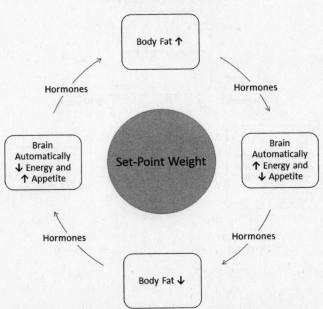

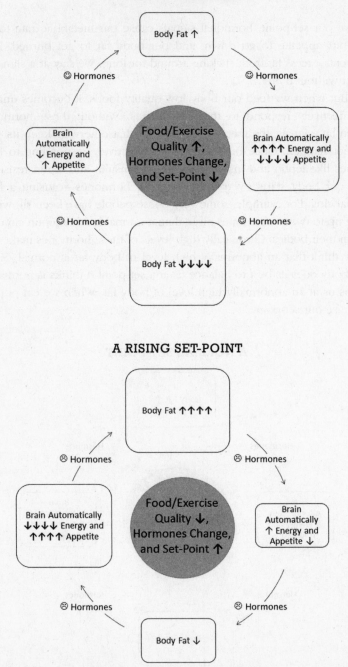

A FALLING SET-POINT

Body Fat ↑

☺ Hormones

☺ Hormones

Brain Automatically ↓ Energy and ↑ Appetite

Food/Exercise Quality ↑, Hormones Change, and Set-Point ↓

Brain Automatically ↑↑↑↑ Energy and ↓↓↓ Appetite

☺ Hormones

☺ Hormones

Body Fat ↓↓↓↓

A RISING SET-POINT

Body Fat ↑↑↑↑

☹ Hormones

☹ Hormones

Brain Automatically ↓↓↓↓ Energy and ↑↑↑↑ Appetite

Food/Exercise Quality ↓, Hormones Change, and Set-Point ↑

Brain Automatically ↑ Energy and Appetite ↓

☹ Hormones

☹ Hormones

Body Fat ↓

HOW TO LOWER YOUR SET-POINT WEIGHT

You may be thinking to yourself: "This set-point science is all well and good, but what about people who lose weight by eating less and exercising more?" Our set-point doesn't mean that it's impossible to lower our body weight by eating less and exercising more or that it's impossible to raise our body weight by doing the opposite. We can do all sorts of unhealthy things to temporarily stray from set-points in the short term. As I noted earlier, we could sit in an ice bath for as long as we can tolerate, and it would temporarily lower our body temperature just as starving as long as we can tolerate will temporarily lower our body weight. However, the set-point wins out over the *long term*. It shows why we have such a hard time *keeping* weight off when we focus on calorie counting. We can absolutely stray from our body weight set-point temporarily via food and exercise *quantity*, but we cannot adjust our set-point itself unless we change the *quality* of our food and exercise. The higher the quality, the lower our set-point.

Consider a nutritional study performed on rats conducted at Penn State University by Barbara Rolls, PhD, chair of Nutritional Sciences.[16] The rats were divided into two groups:

Low-Quality Group: Rats with access to unlimited low- and normal-quality food.
High-Quality Group: Rats with access to unlimited higher-quality food.

As expected, the Low-Quality Group gained weight and the High-Quality Group did not. But here is where the study gets interesting: After the Low-Quality Group became heavy, Rolls took the low-quality food (processed starches and sweets such as such as chips, cookies, and crackers) away from them. Now both the overweight Low-Quality Group and the regular-weight High-Quality Group had access to the same food. The Low-Quality Group, though, stayed at their heavy weight.

Wait a second. How can the same diet keep one group of rats heavy and keep another group slim? Because the Low-Quality Group had changed their set-points.*

---

* Note: We are going to cover a lot of rat or mouse studies. These studies are useful because they allow researchers to do things they could never do on humans and

The High-Quality Group started with a normal set-point and remained at a normal set-point, thanks to a diet of whole, nutritious foods, and therefore maintained a normal weight. The Low-Quality group started with a normal set-point, increased their set-point thanks to a low-quality diet, and thereafter stayed at their heavy weight. Rolls attributed the change in the obese rats to "a long-lasting endocrine or metabolic change."[17] In other words, hormonal clog.

The study gets even more interesting. Rolls then took half of the heavy Low-Quality Group and fed them a diet of only higher-quality food, but much less of it. In other words, she made the heavy rats eat less. Lowering the *quantity* of food caused the rats to *temporarily* lose weight. However, as soon as Rolls stopped starving the Low-Quality Group, they returned to the heavy weight targeted by their recently raised set-point. They did not return to a standard rat weight. The low-quality food they ate at the start of the study raised their set-point and put them on a path of long-term weight gain.

THE IMPACT OF LOW-QUALITY FOOD IN ROLLS'S STUDY

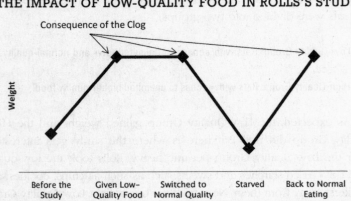

Rolls's study shows us that a steady diet of low-quality food can cause our set-point to rise—which is unsettling news for anyone who's been eating the standard American diet for any length of time. But

because they enable us to eliminate variables like emotions and social pressure. When we observe animal models, we're looking at mammalian biology plain and simple.

here's the good news: studies from all around the world offer evidence that the metabolic and hormonal consequences of eating a low-quality diet are reversible.[18] In their lead article "Neurobiology of Nutrition and Obesity" in the journal *Nutrition Reviews*, Pennington Biomedical Research Center researchers Christopher D. Morrison, PhD, and Hans-Rudolf Berthoud, PhD, noted that "diet-induced leptin resistance," or the dysregulation of one of our key hormones in regulating weight control, "is fully reversible" in genetically identical mice.[19] University of Washington researchers have also discovered that enjoying more whole-food fats—especially natural foods high in omega-3 fats such as salmon, flax seeds, and chia seeds—in place of refined, processed vegetable oils found in starch- and sugar-based junk food, reduces the inflammation in the brain that contributes to an elevated set-point.[20] Additional studies go on to show that 80 percent of individuals with severe insulin resistance—another major factor of set-point elevation—can reverse the damage caused by an overload of sugar and make their cells more sensitive to insulin again by eating a higher-quality diet and exercising smarter.[21] Finally, startling studies out of the Metabolism and Nutrition Research Group at the Université Catholique de Louvain in Belgium prove that when mice were fed a nutritious diet that restored their microbiomes, or healthy gut bacteria, the mice had "markedly improved glucose tolerance, reduced body weight and fat mass, and increased muscle mass," without any changes in the *quantity* of calories they consumed.[22]

In each of these studies, the researchers were able to reset the set-point of mice by changing the *kinds of foods* the mice were fed—not the quantity of what they were fed. In their own words, they were able to reverse "diet-induced metabolic disorders, including fat-mass gain, metabolic endotoxemia [inflammation], adipose tissue inflammation, and insulin resistance."[23] The data are clear: by increasing the quality of our eating and exercise, we can resensitize ourselves to fat-burning hormones, reduce inflammation, and enjoy a metabolism more like that of a naturally thin person.

We know from Dr. Rolls's study that rats that were fed low-quality food ended up with higher set-points. But what about the impact of exercise? Wouldn't rats that exercised more be able to lower even their elevated set-points?

The University of Utah's Dr. Jeffrey Peck devised a test similar to Rolls's study, dividing healthy rats into three groups.[24] First, he looked at the impact of diet on set-point. Each group could eat an unlimited quantity of calories. The only difference was the quality of the calories.

High-Quality Group: Rats with access to unlimited high-quality food.

Low-Quality Group: Rats with access to unlimited low-quality food.

Quinine Group: Rats with access to unlimited food with a bitter substance called quinine added to it.

As expected, the High-Quality Group maintained a standard weight, the Low-Quality Group gained weight, and the Quinine Group lost weight. Peck then made each group of rats eat less of their type of food. All the rats temporarily lost about 10 percent of their body weight.

Peck then stopped starving the rats and they all went back to eating an unlimited amount of their chosen food. The High-Quality Group automatically returned to their standard rat weight. The Low-Quality Group automatically returned to their heavier weight. And the Quinine Group automatically returned to their reduced weight. As in Rolls's study, after eating less, all the rats automatically regained weight, but how much they regained depended on their set-point, which was determined by the quality of their diet. In other words, food *quantity* temporarily moved them away from their set-point, but food *quality* determined the set-point itself.

Next, Peck wanted to explore the effects of exercise on these three groups, so he had his furry subjects burn calories by shivering away all day in a very cold room. All the rats automatically increased how much they ate to offset how much they exercised. Burning more calories simply made the rats eat more calories. Their set-point was un-changed.

Peck then freed the rats from the cold conditions, but continued the experiment. He kept all the groups on their respective diets while feeding them additional calories through a stomach tube. He wanted to see if a higher *quantity* of the same *quality* of calories would have an impact on the rats' set-points. It did not. All the rats automatically adjusted the amount of high-quality, low-quality, or bitter food they ate in order to maintain the normal, higher, or lower weights targeted by their set-points.

Eating less did not cause long-term weight loss. The set-point won. Exercising more did not cause long-term weight loss. The set-point won. Having additional calories pumped directly into the stomach did not cause long-term weight gain. The set-point won. The only factor that did have an impact on rats' long-term weight was the quality of their calories. That worked because it reduced inflammation, resensitized receptors, reregulated hormones, and therefore changed their set-point. Fortunately, recent research reveals a more enjoyable way of changing the quality of our diet and lowering our set-point. (No quinine-laced food for us.) Pablo J. Enriori, PhD, of the Division of Neuroscience at Oregon Health and Science University, has since published a study in the journal *Cell Metabolism* (March 2007) showing that returning mammals to the higher-quality diet they are genetically adapted to reverses the clogging and resulting raised set-point caused by a low-quality eating.

One more study proves this point. In Nancy Rothwell's study at St. George's Hospital Medical School in London, growing rats were divided into Low-Quality American Diet and High-Quality Natural Rat Diet groups.[25] Rothwell let all the growing rats eat as much as they wanted for sixteen days. Keep in mind that both groups should gain weight, as they are young, quickly growing rats. On the seventeenth day the rats continued eating as much as they wanted, but Rothwell

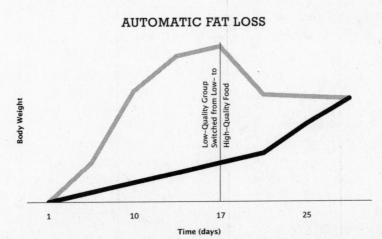

AUTOMATIC FAT LOSS

Body Weight

Low-Quality Group Switched from Low- to High-Quality Food

Time (days)

1 10 17 25

switched the Low-Quality American Diet rats to the High-Quality Natural Rat Diet. Here is what happened (as illustrated in the graph on the preceding page):

The young rats that were becoming obese quickly dropped all their excess weight automatically when the *quality* of their diet improved. The increased quality of their food readjusted their hormones; decreased neurological, digestive, and nervous inflammation; resensitized cells; and lowered their set-point. We can do the same once we stop focusing on quantity and start applying the science of quality.

Let's look at the four major problems of the traditional quantity-focused fat-loss approach:

1. Eating less does *not* cause long-term fat loss.
2. Exercising more does *not* cause long-term fat loss.
3. Exercising less does *not* cause long-term fat gain.
4. Eating more does *not* cause long-term fat gain.

In the next few chapters we'll look at what scientists have to say about each of these statements. They already know the answers and they can prove it. That's good for us, because by knowing the facts, we can finally start to burn fat and protect our health permanently.

Eating More Doesn't Make You Fat

Let's imagine a world where calorie counting and eating less of the traditional Western diet are actually the keys to long-term fat loss. Now let's try an experiment. We'll divide a group of people in half. We'll feed one half 120 fewer calories per day for eight years. What would happen? If weight was ruled by conventional calorie counting, the math would be pretty easy. Multiply 120 fewer calories per day times 365 days in a year, times eight years, and the total equals 350,400 fewer calories. Take that sum and divide it by the 3,500 calories in a pound of body fat, and math tells us that these people should have avoided gaining 100 pounds compared with the other group. The math is easy, but it's incorrect.

Instead, let's look at a real-life study: the Women's Health Initiative, a study that tracked nearly 49,000 women for eight years.[26] Just as in our experiment, the women in one group ate an average of 120 fewer calories a day than the other group. Remember, that adds up to 350,400 fewer calories. How much lighter was the average woman who ate 350,400 fewer calories?

The answer: 0.88 pound.

That is not a typo. Eating 350,400 fewer calories had less than 1 percent of the impact predicted by calorie math. Eating less of a traditional Western diet does not cause long-term fat loss because this approach incorrectly assumes that taking in fewer calories forces our body to burn fat. That has been clinically proved to be false. Eating less does not force us to burn body fat. It forces us to burn fewer calories. That is why dieters walk around tired and crabby all day. Their bodies and brains have slowed down.

When our body needs calories and none are around, it is forced to make a decision: go through all the hassle of converting calories from body fat or just slow down on burning calories. Given the choice, slowing down wins. Even worse, if we still don't have enough energy, our body burns muscle, not fat. Studies show that up to 70 percent of the nonwater weight lost when people are eating less comes from burning muscle—not body fat. Only after it's cannibalized this muscle will our body burn fat.

Want to set someone up to be fatter and sicker in the long run? Slow down her metabolism and take away her muscle tissue. As soon as she gets tired of being hungry and feeling terrible all day every day, she will go back to eating a normal amount of calories but need fewer of them thanks to her slowed-down metabolism and missing muscle. Now her body sees eating a normal amount as overeating and creates new body fat.

In the *Journal of the American Medical Association*, George L. Thorpe, MD, a physician within the American Medical Association itself, wrote that eating less makes us lose weight, not "by selective reduction of adipose deposits [body fat], but by wasting of all body tissues . . . therefore, any success obtained must be maintained by chronic undernourishment."[27] It is not practical or healthy to keep ourselves "chronically under-nourished," so we don't. Instead, we yo-yo diet. The standard approach to fat loss we've all been taught sets us up for long-term fat gain, not fat loss.

Why does our body behave this way? When we do not provide our body with enough essential nutrients (vitamins, minerals, and essential fatty and amino acids) our body goes into "starvation mode." What does our body want more of when it thinks we are starving? Stored energy. What is a great source of stored energy? Body fat. So when our body thinks we are starving, does it want to get rid of or hold on to body fat? It wants to hold on. What does our body want less of when we are starving? It wants less metabolically active tissue. What type of tissue burns a lot of calories? Muscle tissue. So when our body thinks we are starving, it gets rid of calorie-hungry muscle tissue.

The research is clear: if we want to burn fat and boost our health for the next sixty years as opposed to the next sixty days, let's not starve ourselves. Think about it like this: Imagine you're watching TV and you see a commercial for a new medication. The ad tells you the medication slightly improves your vision as long as you keep yourself

Don't the Laws of Thermodynamics Prove Eating Less Burns Body Fat?

> The principle that weight gain [depends only on calorie quantity] would violate the second law of thermodynamics.
>
> —Richard Feinman, PhD, professor of biochemistry,
> State University of New York Health Science Center[28]

We know the traditional approach to fat loss fails more than 95 percent of the time, yet common sense seems to tell us, "If you eat less and exercise more, you must burn body fat. Anything else violates the laws of thermodynamics."

There are four laws of thermodynamics. The two that apply to burning body fat do not prove that reducing the number of calories eaten makes the body burn fat. They tell us energy cannot be created or destroyed; energy can only change forms. When people eat less, the body must do *something*. That's it. The applicable laws of thermodynamics prove nothing about *what* the body must do.

Remember how it is easier for your metabolism to slow down than to burn body fat? And remember how it makes more sense to burn calorie-hungry muscle than it does to burn protective body fat? Put those two facts together and, instead of proving that eating less equals long-term fat loss, the applicable laws of thermodynamics prove that eating less makes the body slow down and burn muscle, which leads to long-term fat gain—not fat loss.

The relevant question isn't "Can we manually regulate body fat by eating less and exercising more?" That's like asking, "Can we manually regulate blood sugar by injecting insulin?" Why is anyone talking about taking over basic functions within broken bodies before asking, "What is breaking our body?" Let's heal the body instead of struggling through life with a broken one.

chronically sleep-deprived. At the end of the commercial, a quieter voice lists the medication's long-term side effects. One of them is that your vision will become much worse if you ever go back to getting a good night's sleep. Would you ever use that medication?

Of course not. You can't go through life exhausted. The temporary benefit isn't worth the long-term side effects. Sadly, millions of people fall victim to the exhausting side effects of starvation dieting every day.

THE SIDE EFFECTS OF EATING LESS

My favorite experiment that demonstrates the side effects of starvation dieting took place at the University of Geneva and involved three groups of rats all eating the same quality of food.

1. Normal Group: Adult rats eating normally
2. Eat Less Group: Adult rats temporarily losing weight by eating less
3. Naturally Skinny Group: Young rats who naturally weighed about as much as the adult Eat Less Group immediately after the adult rats were starved

If the study were conducted on humans, the Normal Group would be typical thirty-five-year-old women. The Eat Less Group would be thirty-five-year-old women cutting calories until they fit into their high school jeans. And the Naturally Skinny Group would be high school girls who fit into size four jeans without trying.

For the first ten days of the study, the Eat Less Group ate 50 percent less than usual while the Normal Group ate normally. On the tenth day

1. The Normal Group kept eating normally.
2. The Eat Less Group stopped starving themselves and started eating normally.
3. The Naturally Skinny Group ate normally.

This went on for twenty-five days and the study ended on day thirty-five.

At the end of the thirty-five-day study, the Normal Group had eaten normally for thirty-five days. The Eat Less Group had eaten less for ten

SETUP OF THE UNIVERSITY OF GENEVA STUDY

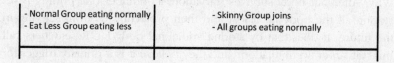

- Normal Group eating normally
- Eat Less Group eating less

- Skinny Group joins
- All groups eating normally

Day 1   **Day 10**   **Day 35**

days and then normally for twenty-five days. And the Naturally Skinny Group had eaten normally for twenty-five days.

Which group do you think weighed the most and had the highest body fat percentage at the end? The Naturally Skinny Group seems like an easy "no," since these rats are younger and naturally thinner than the other rats. Traditional fat-loss theory would say the Eat Less Group is an easy "no" as well, since these rats ate 50 percent less for ten days. So the Normal Group weighed the most and had the highest body fat percentage at the end of the study, right?

Surprisingly, no.

The Eat Less Group weighed the most and had the highest percent body fat. Even though they ate less for ten days, they were significantly heavier than those who ate normally all the way through. Eating less caused metabolic adjustments that led the rats to gain—not lose—body fat.

Here are the data:

A SIDE EFFECT OF STARVATION

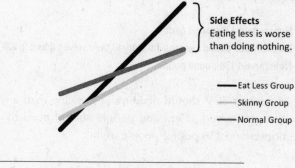

Side Effects
Eating less is worse
than doing nothing.

Weight

Eat Less Group
Skinny Group
Normal Group

Day 10   Day 35

Talk about side effects. Eating less was worse than doing nothing. Why? After our body survives starvation, its number one priority is restoring all the body fat it lost and then protecting us from starving in the future. It does that by storing additional body fat. Researchers call this "fat super accumulation," and they believe it is a primary trigger for "relapsing obesity"—also known as yo-yo dieting.[29]

The most disturbing aspect of fat super accumulation is that it does not require us to eat a lot. All we have to do is go back to eating a normal amount. The Eat Less Group in the study gained a massive amount of body fat quickly while eating *the same amount* as the Normal Group and the Naturally Skinny Group. Why? The body was trying to make up for the past losses.

Eating less also slowed the metabolism. Subject a slowed-down metabolism to the exact same food and exercise and out comes more body fat. The University of Geneva researchers reported that the Eat Less Group's metabolisms were burning body fat over 500 percent less efficiently and had slowed down by 15 percent by the end of the study.

For another example of starvation's long-term side effects, consider a study conducted by Dr. Rudolph Leibel, director of the Division of Molecular Genetics in the Department of Pediatrics at Columbia University Medical Center.[30] A group of people weighing an average of 335 pounds starved themselves down to 220 pounds. After the period of extreme calorie restriction ended, the researchers wanted to see what impact eating less had on the 220-pound dieters' need to burn body fat. To do this they brought in people who were the same age but naturally slim. This gave the researchers three groups of people to compare:

1. Nonstarved 335-pound people
2. Formerly 335-pound people who starved themselves down to 220 pounds
3. Nonstarved 138-pound people

Just as a larger SUV should need more gasoline than a smaller motorcycle, the nonstarved 335-pound people should need more calories than the nonstarved 138-pound people, right?

Yes.

All things being equal, more body weight means more calories

CALORIES NEEDED PER DAY

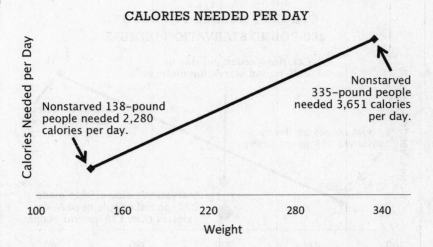

Nonstarved 138-pound people needed 2,280 calories per day.

Nonstarved 335-pound people needed 3,651 calories per day.

needed per day to maintain and move more mass. So you would think that after losing 115 pounds, the 220-pound people slid right down the graph. Right?

CALORIES NEEDED PER DAY

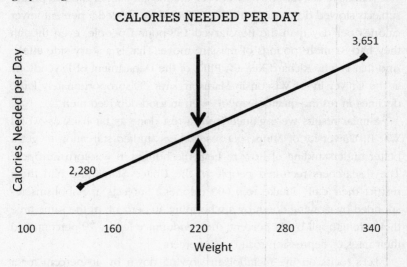

Not necessarily. It depends on how the 115 pounds were lost. After all, we know that starvation burns calorie-hungry muscle while slowing down the metabolism. So, how many calories did the 220-pound starvation dieters need after having starved away 115 pounds?

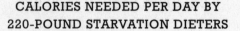

CALORIES NEEDED PER DAY BY
220-POUND STARVATION DIETERS

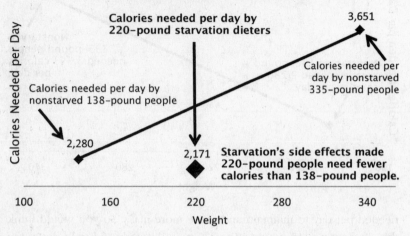

Thanks to starvation's side effects, the metabolism of the 220-pound subjects slowed down dramatically. In fact, they needed 5 percent fewer calories per day than the nonstarved 138-pound people, even though they had 82 more pounds of mass to move. That is a scary side effect. And that is why Richard Keesey, PhD, of the Department of Psychology at the University of Wisconsin-Madison, says, "Disproportionately large declines in resting metabolism are seen in food-deprived men."[31]

Similar results were gained from a test done as far back as World War II. University of Minnesota researchers studied starvation to get a better understanding of how to help the hungry in war-torn Europe.[32] The researchers recruited people in the United States and had them restrict their daily intake to 1,600 calories.* Subjects' metabolisms responded by slowing down by a whopping 40 percent. At the same time their strength fell by 28 percent, their endurance fell by 79 percent, and their rates of depression rose by 36 percent.

Let's focus on the metabolism slowing down by 40 percent for a moment. Say Jillian needs and eats 2,000 calories per day. But now

---

* Sixteen hundred calories per day is considered generous by today's "eat less" advocates.

Jillian wants to drop a few pounds for her vacation in two weeks, so she reads a magazine that tells her to starve herself and she cuts back to 1,600 calories per day. According to this study, Jillian's metabolism would slow down by 40 percent and she would need only 1,200 calories per day. Before Jillian ate less, she needed 2,000 calories per day and ate 2,000 per day. After eating less, Jillian needed only 1,200 calories per day but ate 1,600 per day. When she stops eating less, she will eat 2,000 calories per day while needing only 1,200 per day. That's not helpful.

In addition to being deprived of their need to burn body fat, as soon as the World War II study subjects stopped eating less, thanks to their set-point, they ate an average of 5,000 calories a day until they gained all the weight they lost back plus 5 percent. That is the good news. The bad news is that their body fat percentage was 52 percent higher than before they starved themselves. All the muscle they burned was replaced by body fat. They experienced fat super accumulation.

THE MORE WE STARVE OURSELVES, THE WORSE OFF WE ARE

Attempting to eat less of a traditional Western diet is counterproductive because it leads to yo-yo dieting, and yo-yo dieting increases our risk of heart attack, stroke, diabetes, high blood pressure, cancer, immune system failure, eating disorders, impaired cognitive function, chronic fatigue, and depression. If that's not bad enough, the more often we yo-yo, the easier it is to yo-yo for the rest of our lives. "It is only the rate of weight regain, not the fact of weight regain, that appears open to debate," says David Garner, PhD, professor of psychiatry at Michigan State University.[33]

In a University of Pennsylvania study, rats yo-yoed up, down, back up, back down, and then back up.[34] The second time the rats tried to lose weight by eating less, they lost weight 100 percent more slowly and regained the weight 300 percent faster than the first time they ate less. The rats who yo-yoed the second time stored food as body fat 400 percent more efficiently than rats who constantly ate a fattening diet.

Doing nothing is better than just eating less of the traditional Western diet. This study shows it is 400 percent better.

However, even after all this evidence, there still may be a voice in the back of your head saying, "Now hold on. There has to be some truth in 'eating less means less body fat,' because that's what everybody says." I felt the same way. Then I discovered a Harvard study of 67,272 people.[35] The researchers divided this large sample into five groups according to the quantity of calories they ate and found that the *less* people ate, the *more* body fat they had. This finding is shown in the following chart, where "Body Mass Index" approximates "body fat."*

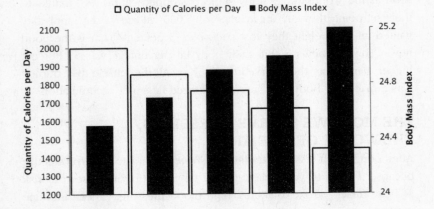

LOWER CALORIES, HIGHER BMI

☐ Quantity of Calories per Day ■ Body Mass Index

Hunger is not healthy. Think about starving yourself to burn fat; it's like drinking salt water to quench your thirst. Both seem as if they should be helpful and they both provide some relief in the short term, but both do more harm than good in the long term. University of California researchers say, "There is little support for the notion that diets lead to lasting weight loss or health benefits."[36] University of Washington researchers say, "Energy-restricted diets are a physiologically unsound means to achieve weight reduction."[37] Starvation does not make

* From the Centers for Disease Control and Prevention: "Body Mass Index (BMI) is a number calculated from a person's weight and height. BMI provides a reliable indicator of body fatness for most people and is used to screen for weight categories that may lead to health problems." (Source: http://www.cdc.gov/healthyweight/assessing/bmi.)

us thin. It makes us stocky, sick, and sad. It's bad for health and it's bad for fat loss.

EAT MORE, BURN MORE

Eating more low-quality processed foods causes us to gain body fat. But that does not mean eating more high-quality whole foods produces the same result. Interestingly enough, eating more of the right foods has been clinically proved to help us burn fat over the long term. Consider the evidence:

- A study at the University of Connecticut found that people in the eat-more-high-quality-food group ate 300 more calories *per day* and burned more body fat.[38]
- A study at the University of Pennsylvania found that people in the eat-more-high-quality-food group ate a total of 9,500 more calories *over six months* and lost 200 percent more weight.[39]
- A study published in *Obesity Research* found that people in the eat-more-high-quality-food group ate a total of 25,000 more calories *over three months* without gaining any additional weight.[40]
- A study published in the *Journal of Adolescent Health* found that people in the eat-more-high-quality-food group ate a total of 65,000 more calories *over four months* and lost 141 percent more weight.[41]

How are these results possible? Research suggests two main reasons: First, a calorie is *not* merely a calorie (more on that soon). Second, more in means more out—only as long as we're unclogged. Let's look at how hormonally healing ourselves enables us to restore our natural set-point and to burn—instead of store—excess calories.

Researchers at the Mayo Clinic fed people 1,000 extra calories per day for eight weeks.[42] A thousand extra calories per day for eight weeks totals 56,000 extra calories. Nobody gained sixteen pounds—56,000 calories' worth—of body fat. The most anyone gained was a little over half that. The least anyone gained was basically nothing—less than a pound.

How could that be true? People ate an additional 56,000 calories and gained basically zero body fat? How can 56,000 extra calories add up to nothing?

That's because extra calories don't have to turn into body fat. They could be burned off automatically. The medical journal *QJM* reports, "Food in excess of immediate requirements . . . can easily be disposed of, being burnt up and dissipated as heat. Did this capacity not exist, obesity would be almost universal."[43]

Eating more and gaining less is possible because when we're hormonally healthy, we have all sorts of underappreciated ways to deal with calories other than storing them as body fat. In the Mayo Clinic study, researchers measured three of them:

1. Increase the amount of calories burned daily.
2. Increase the amount of calories burned digesting food.
3. Increase the amount calories burned via unconscious activity.

Here is what they found:

Daily Response to 1,000 Extra Calories

	Clogged	Unclogged
Base Calories Burned Daily	Decreased by 100 calories ☹	Increased by 360 calories ☺
Calories Burned Digesting Food	Increased by 28 calories ☺	Increased by 256 calories ☺
Calories Burned via Unconscious Activity	Decreased by 98 calories ☹	Increased by 692 calories ☺☺
Total Daily Response	**Burned 170 Fewer Calories** ☹	**Burned 1,308 More Calories** ☺☺☺

That is how some people ate 56,000 extra calories and instead of storing the excess calories as body fat, gained virtually no weight. A lower set-point does its best to automatically balance more calories in with more calories out by upping the calories we burn keeping ourselves alive and digesting food, and via unconscious activity.

There is no shortage of proof. Take a study performed by researchers at Harvard Medical School and King's College, London University. Students were divided into two groups according to the "ease with which they maintained a relatively lean body weight."[44] The researchers called the group that maintained their weight without trying "lean." I call them unclogged. The researchers called the students who struggled with their weight "postobese." I call them clogged.

While participants in both groups were similar in age, gender, size, and activity level, and all maintained a steady body weight throughout the study, their metabolic profiles varied in two major ways. First, the students who struggled with their weight actually ate less than their effortlessly lean counterparts "by 30 percent per kilogram of body weight." Second, the unclogged students automatically burned more than 500 additional calories per day compared with their clogged peers. In other words, the unclogged students *ate significantly more and burned significantly more* than the clogged students, all factors being equal.

The study doesn't stop there. The researchers then went on to feed all the participants 300-calorie meals and discovered that "the overall thermogenic [calorie burning] response of the [clogged] subjects to the 300 calorie meal was only half that measure in the [unclogged] subjects." Again, when they ate more, the unclogged participants automatically burned more and the clogged participants automatically stored more. The researchers concluded, "These findings provide further evidence for a subnormal thermogenic [calorie burning] response to food in those with a predisposition to obesity." Clogged individuals do not gain weight because they eat a lot and exercise too little. This and many other studies show that overweight people eat significantly fewer calories and are as active as naturally thin people. This is not an issue of gluttony or laziness. The issue is biology: Their bodies have lost their natural ability to stay slim, to burn more when they eat more. It's not a moral issue. It's not a willpower issue. It's a metabolic issue.

We know that the weight-loss advice we commonly read in books and see in the media isn't helping us. Eating less of the standard American diet and doing more of a traditional exercise program doesn't cause long-term weight loss. So where can we turn? There must be an institution that can provide us with reliable information on health and weight loss. How about our own government guidelines and regulations?

Sadly, the information coming out of government institutions isn't as reliable as you might think. In fact, the very people responsible for teaching us about eating and exercise—the United States Department of Agriculture (USDA)—don't seem to be up on the latest science. Take this excerpt from chapter 3 of the USDA's *Dietary Guidelines for Ameri-*

cans: "Since many adults gain weight slowly over time, even small decreases in calorie intake can help avoid weight gain."[45]

If "small decreases in calorie intake" lead to gradual weight loss, does that mean "small decreases in calorie intake" will eventually make us weigh nothing? Of course not. Why? Because we're dealing with biology, not math. But if that is true, then how can a small decrease in calorie intake help us practically avoid weight gain long term?

It can't.

The issue is not that our body wants us to weigh less but that too many calories per day are blocking it. The issue is that our body does not want us to weigh less thanks to our elevated set-point. The same mechanism preventing "small decreases in calorie intake" from making you weigh nothing (your set-point) also prevents your body from burning off excess fat effectively right now.

When you think about how hard every living organism works to maintain balance, our set-point weight makes perfect sense. What doesn't make sense is the advice of many respected health institutions on this topic, such as the American Heart Association, which advises, "How can you manage your weight in a healthful way? The answer is simple: balance the calories you take in with the calories you burn."[46] That advice is especially troubling since the AHA also published a piece in its journal, *Circulation*, noting, "Few reliable data are available on the relative contributions to this obesity epidemic by energy intake and energy expenditure."[47] If "few reliable data are available," then what is the basis for its recommendations?

Here's what the data actually show. Harvard researchers looked at the eating patterns of more than 50,000 people, divided into fifths, according to the quantity and quality of calories they ate.[48] This large sample demonstrated two points:

1. Eating more correlated with less body fat.
2. Higher-quality food correlated with less body fat.

If we can escape the trap of old calorie-quantity (versus calorie-quality) myths, we will never have to worry about our weight again. Now let's take a look at how we can increase the quality of our exercise to start burning more fat in less time.

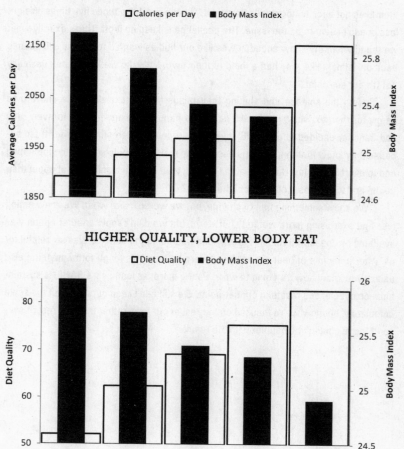

MORE FOOD, LESS BODY FAT

☐ Calories per Day ■ Body Mass Index

HIGHER QUALITY, LOWER BODY FAT

☐ Diet Quality ■ Body Mass Index

From Short-Term Weight Loss to Long-Term Health:
Jay and Jennifer Jacobs's Story

Jay and Jennifer Jacobs inspired a nation with their nearly 300-pound combined weight loss while on NBC's *Biggest Loser*. While they were thrilled with the results they got from dedicating every hour of their lives to calorie counting and extreme exercise, Jay and Jennifer knew they had to find a more sustainable approach once their lives got back to normal. As Jay put it, "I have lost 100 pounds five times. Weight loss doesn't seem to be the issue. The challenge is keeping it off. That's exactly what we found when the show ended. It was like our bodies wanted to put the 300 pounds back on. Almost like they had a mind of their own. Little did we know, they basically do! It's our set-point."

Seeing the science and shifting their minds from "make the scale and crowd happy for the next show" to "make ourselves happy, slim, and healthy forever," Jay and Jennifer decided to go SANE. It was a particularly interesting shift for them because they know firsthand that the best way to make the scale smile is to stop eating and to exercise all day. But what about making their set-point smile? What about their health and waistlines for the rest of their lives?

"We knew something had to change, but we weren't sure what. We knew eating less and exercising more worked short-term, but we didn't know another option was available for the long term. This is why understanding the science was so helpful for us. After a lifetime of hearing 'eat less, exercise more' it's tough to try anything else unless you know how it's going to work. Eating more, as long as it's SANE, is sustainable, enjoyable, and resetting our set-point. We still can't keep ourselves off the scale completely, but now we're focused on the rest of our lives rather than the rest of season 11, and couldn't be happier with the results."

Exercising More Doesn't Make You Thin

We have seen that eating less is not effective. But what about doing more aerobic exercise? From the perspective of our body, there is basically no difference between the two. More calories out is effectively the same as fewer calories in. Everything that makes the "eat less" principle fail long term makes "exercise more" fail long term too.

Now, I'm not saying that all exercise is pointless. What is ineffective is traditional high-impact and moderate-intensity exercise like jogging. Low-impact and low-intensity activity such as walking is phenomenal for our health. No-impact and high-intensity activity such as eccentric resistance training is instrumental in lowering our set-point. We'll cover that science later, but first we have to free our minds from the conventional "jog more to burn more" mythology.

In the same way that people drink more water when they exercise more, they also eat more when they exercise more. In his textbook, *Obesity and Leanness*, Hugo Rony, MD, of Northwestern University, notes, "Consistently high or low energy expenditures result in consistently high or low levels of appetite. Thus men doing heavy physical work spontaneously eat more than men engaged in sedentary occupations."[49] Jeffrey M. Friedman, MD, PhD, head of the Laboratory of Molecular Genetics at Rockefeller University in New York, makes a similar point: "Exercise by itself has not been shown to be highly effective in treating obesity because the increased energy use from exercise is generally offset by increased caloric intake."[50]

Compounding the problem, many people who exercise more do not eat high-quality food; they get the majority of their calories from low-quality starches and sweeteners. Therefore, for most people, exercising more triggers the consumption of more low-quality food. More *low-quality* food means more hormonal clogging and a higher setpoint. Far from burning body fat, we burn time and build up clogs.

Timothy Church, MD, MPH, PhD, who is with the Exercise Biology Laboratory at Pennington Biomedical Research Center, worked with a group of overweight college-age women to burn 2,000 calories a week through exercise for eighteen months and found that the women experienced *no* weight loss. Church divided the women into four groups:

1. No change in exercise
2. Exercise more
3. Exercise even more
4. Exercise way more

After six months, there was no statistically different change in body fat across the groups. Church notes that more exercise did not cause more body fat to be burned because "a relatively high dose of exercise results in *compensatory* mechanisms that attenuate [offset] weight loss."[51] He points out that most exercise guidelines for weight loss recommend two hundred to three hundred minutes per week, but they found this amount of exercise induces compensation that results in *significantly less* weight loss than predicted. Marathoner Kim Raine captures a more typical experience: "I've run eighteen marathons and I put one pound on for each one. Eighteen marathons and eighteen pounds heavier. It is so maddening."[52]

Here is a best case "exercising more" scenario: Michelle goes for a thirty-minute jog and burns 170 more calories than she would have burned by sitting at home and reading this book. She is trying hard to cut calories, so she does not drink any sugary sports drinks and fights through the hunger pangs after her jog. At dinner Michelle unconsciously drinks an extra glass of low-fat milk thanks to her increased thirst and hunger. The net result of her jog is thirteen more calories than if she had not exercised. Thanks to her set-point, the 13 extra calories don't matter, but if Michelle knew what was really going on, she could probably find something more productive to do with that thirty minutes.

30 min. jog	−170 calories
12 oz. milk	+183 calories
Net	+13 calories

It's much easier to eat calories than it is to burn calories, so more commonly, people will have a sweetened sports drink while pounding it out on the treadmill. Afterward, they easily overeat low-quality food. The net result is more low-quality food and a higher set-point.

30 min. jog	−170 calories
24 oz. sports drink	+189 calories
Extra half serving of fettuccine Alfredo	+390 calories
Net	+409 hormonally clogging calories

The food industry is well aware that exercising more encourages eating more low-quality food. The list below shows food companies who serve on the executive board of the American Council on Fitness and Nutrition:

Coca-Cola Company

PepsiCo

Hershey Foods Corporation

Sara Lee Corporation

Kellogg Company

Kraft Foods

General Mills

Campbell Soup Company

ConAgra Foods

Del Monte Foods

Grocery Manufacturers Association

H.J. Heinz Company

Masterfoods USA

National Restaurant Association

Unilever United States

American Association of Advertising Agencies

American Beverage Association

Association of National Advertisers

Are these companies eager to tell us to exercise more because it is good for fat loss or because it is good for business? The National Soft Drink Association advises us to "consume at least eight glasses of fluids daily, *even more when you exercise*. A variety of beverages, *including soft drinks*, can contribute to proper hydration."[53]

But isn't jogging good for our heart? Not when compared with the smarter types of exercise we will cover later. The American Heart Association found that jogging injures more than half of the people who do it. This high injury rate is due in part to the fact that every mile we run, our feet hit the ground about 900 times. Let's say you weigh 150 pounds. That means for every mile you run, you are smashing 135,000 pounds of force against your joints, ligaments, and every other part of your body. You could say that's like dropping thirty-seven Toyota Camrys on yourself every time you go for a jog. Jogging is "healthy exercise" in the same way that boxing is "healthy exercise."

But doesn't traditional exercise help relieve stress and make us feel good? Maybe, but we'll see that there are plently of other ways to de-stress and stay active without any unhealthy side effects.

The theory that we have an obesity epidemic because people are not exercising enough is disproved by the data. In a July 2013 report, the Institute for Health Metrics and Evaluation found, "As physical activity increased between 2001 and 2009, so did the percentage of the population considered obese."[54] Other studies go on to show that obese people do about the same amount of physical activity as lean people do.[55]

The only "weight versus activity" relationship that has been proved is that obesity may lead to inactivity. Consider the conclusion of a 2004 University of Copenhagen study: "This study did *not* support that physical inactivity . . . is associated with the development of obesity, but . . . that obesity may lead to physical inactivity."[56] More body fat may lead to less exercise, not the other way around. As Dr. Brad Metcalf, a researcher in the Department of Endocrinology and Metabolism at the Peninsula Medical School, concluded in his 2011 study: "Physical inactivity appears to be the result of fatness rather than its cause. This reverse causality may explain why attempts to tackle childhood obesity by promoting physical activity have been largely unsuccessful."[57]

It's helpful to compare the idea that "exercising less causes obesity" to the idea that "partying less causes aging." People party less when they become older. They do not get older because they are partying less. With age come metabolic changes that make staying out until 3 a.m. harder. The same holds true with exercise and obesity. People may exercise less because they are obese. They do not become obese because they are exercising less. With obesity come deep metabolic changes that make exercise harder.

Also, common sense tells us that if exercising less is the cause of our collective weight issues, we must be collectively exercising less. Are we?

Not even close.

The idea of aerobic exercise did not even exist in the mainstream until the 1968 publication of Dr. Kenneth H. Cooper's book *Aerobics*. Pauline Entin, PhD, associate dean for academic affairs at Northern Arizona University, explains the common view before then: "In the 1930s and '40s . . . high volume endurance training was thought to be bad for the heart. Through the '50s and even '60s, exercise was not thought to be useful . . . and endurance exercise was thought to be harmful to women."[58] During that same period the percentage of obese Americans was dramatically lower than today. Nowadays, Americans do more intentional "exercise" than people anywhere else in the world and make up the sixth-heaviest population in the world. How could doing too little of something that we did even less of before the problem existed cause the problem?

To illustrate the rise of aerobic exercise, between 1972 and 2005 health-club-related revenues have increased an estimated 15,000 percent after adjusting for inflation. The first Boston Marathon in 1964 had 300 runners. In 2009, more than 26,000 people ran. The first New York City marathon in 1970 had 137 entrants. In 2008, about 60,000 entered. As Eric Oliver, PhD, professor of political science at the University of Chicago, tells us, "[Americans] are voluntarily exercising more than ever. . . . While it seems perfectly clear that our lives are less physically demanding than they were in the 1950s, it's not necessarily the case that we are cumulatively burning fewer calories."[59]

Some experts say that we are getting heavier because we are using laborsaving devices. Yet that doesn't match the data either. The vast majority of laborsaving devices became common in households decades before obesity shot up. Use of dishwashers, washing machines, vacuum cleaners, and all the major laborsaving devices increased most between 1945 and 1965. However, obesity increased little during that time period. Use of these devices increased very little between 1978 and 1998 while obesity rates shot up. So how could laborsaving devices be the cause of weight problems?

Digging into the data and abandoning *assumptions* about our activity levels, researchers like New York University's Marion Nestle tell us that "the activity levels of Americans appear to have changed little, if at all, from the 1970s to the 1990s."[60]

What about all the TV watching? That's got to be the cause, right? That too does not correspond with the facts. Tsinghua University professor Seth Roberts determined that "time spent watching TV increased by 45 percent from 1965 to 1975, yet obesity increased little over that time; from 1975 to 1995, when obesity shot up, TV watching increased only a little."[61]

Wait a second. We have to be burning fewer calories than our hunter-gatherer ancestors, right? Unexpectedly, no. A landmark study was published in July 2012 proving that "total energy expenditure is *statistically indistinguishable* between Westerners and Hadza foragers (one of the few remaining hunter-gatherer tribes)."[62] The data show that hunter-gatherers *were* more physically active, but "average daily energy expenditure of traditional Hadza foragers was no different than that of Westerners after controlling for body size." How is this possible? How could hunter-gatherers "exercise more" but burn the same total number of calories as we do?

The hunter-gatherers automatically burned less when they were inactive to make up for burning more when they were active. As the researchers concluded, their results "suggest that physical activity may be only one piece of a dynamic metabolic strategy that is continuously responding to changes in energy availability and demand." What is a "dynamic metabolic strategy"? The set-point.

Finally, if general activity level determined weight, then the thinnest people in the world would be manual laborers, while the heaviest would be desk workers. People with manual jobs are "active" at least forty hours a week, every week, at these jobs. People with desk jobs are "inactive" at least forty hours a week. Are manual laborers slimmer than desk workers?

Let's look at the research. The Centers for Disease Control and Prevention (CDC) collected data from over 68,000 adults and found that obesity *rises* as income falls and manual labor—that is, work-related activity—rises. The data suggest that, on average, active manual laborers are heavier than inactive desk workers. Therefore, it seems that activity level is not a good predictor of fitness.

Now that we've debunked the first Calorie Myth by showing that eating less and exercising more is not the way to get healthy and slim for the long term, let's look at how the second Calorie Myth conspires to undermine your weight-loss efforts.

The Myth That All Calories
Are Created Equal

Our second Calorie Myth is one that is touted in diet books and on television shows, and used in the formulas of many popular weight-loss
programs.

Calorie Myth #2: A Calorie Is a Calorie

Richard Feinman, PhD, of SUNY's Health Science Center, said it
best: "Attacking the obesity epidemic will involve giving up many old
ideas that have not been productive. 'A calorie is a calorie' might be a
good place to start."[63] In order to streamline calorie counting, we've
been told that all calories are created equal. Think about using this
kind of equivocation—which doesn't take quality into account—with
something else that's essential to our health: water. If you were thirsty,
would you stop to drink from a polluted creek or a muddy puddle in
the middle of the road? Of course you wouldn't—because the issue isn't
just about quenching your thirst. You know that water quality matters a
lot. The solution to the puddle problem isn't to "drink less water," but
rather to "drink higher-quality water"; similarly, the solution to today's
obesity epidemic isn't to "eat less food," but rather to "eat higher-quality
food."

THE FOUR CALORIE-QUALITY FACTORS

Beyond battling our basic biology, calorie counting is bound to fail us because not all calories are equal in our bodies.

Calorie counting is rooted in the assumption that our bodies work like balance scales. Balance scales do not measure quality. On a balance scale, a pound of feathers weighs the same as a pound of lead. Quality is irrelevant. So on a balance scale, 300 calories of vegetables is the same as 300 calories of pasta.

The problem is that the body is not a balance scale.

Let's look at the issue another way. Breathing in polluted air for thirty years has a different effect on our respiratory system from breathing in the same quantity of fresh air. In the same fashion, putting 2,000 calories of low-quality food into our metabolic system has a different effect on our weight from putting in the same quantity of high-quality food.

Marshall University conducted a childhood obesity study in which researchers divided obese kids into two groups:

1. Cut Quantity: Kids went on conventional low-calorie diets.
2. Change Quality: Kids went on unlimited-calorie low-carbohydrate diets.

After two months, the Change Quality kids lost eleven pounds, but the Cut Quantity kids *gained* five pounds. We do not have to go on a low-carbohydrate diet, but this study is a great example of how critical calorie quality is. People ate as much as they wanted whenever they wanted and still burned body fat because they changed the quality of their calories.

So how do we know what a "quality" calories is? The quality of our calories can be determined by assessing our food based on four criteria:

1. **S**atiety: how quickly the calories fill us up and how long they keep us full
2. **A**ggression: how likely the calories are to be stored as body fat
3. **N**utrition: how many nutrients—vitamins, minerals, essential fatty acids, essential amino acids—the calories provide
4. **E**fficiency: how many of the calories can be stored as body fat

The more Satisfying, unAggressive, Nutritious, and inEfficient a calorie is, the higher its quality. The more SANE it is. The more it heals our hormones, prevents overeating, and lowers our set-point. Conversely, the more unSatisfying, Aggressive, not Nutritious, and Efficient a calorie is, the lower its quality. The more inSANE it is. The more it harms our hormones, encourages overeating, and raises our set-point. The more we understand the four calorie-quality factors, the more clearly we will see how eating *more* high-quality SANE food is the only practical way to burn fat and boost health long term.

Illustrating the importance of calorie quality, in each of the studies that follow, all the study participants ate the exact same quantity of calories (these are called isocaloric studies), but one group's calories were of much higher quality (were much more SANE) than those of the other groups:

> A review completed at the University of Florida analyzed eighty-seven studies and found that those people who ate SANE calories lost an average of twelve more pounds of body fat compared with those who ate an equal quantity of inSANE calories.[64]
>
> Researchers at Cornell University split people into three groups, each eating 1,800 calories per day, but at different levels of SANEity. The most SANE group lost 86.5 percent more body fat than the least SANE group.[65]
>
> In the *Annals of Internal Medicine*, researchers at the Clinical Investigation Center, US Naval Hospital, compared a reduced-calorie inSANE diet with a reduced-calorie SANE diet. After ten days the SANE diet burned twice as much body fat.[66]
>
> A review published in the journal *Nutrition & Metabolism* covered nine additional trials demonstrating that people who eat SANE calories lose more weight than those who eat the *exact* same quantity of inSANE calories.[67]

Let's look at each of the four factors of SANE eating. We'll start with Satiety (which comes from the same root as *satisfying*).

The Philosophy of Long-Term Fat Loss and Health

The eighteenth-century German philosopher Immanuel Kant proposed a helpful theory for thinking about moral issues: We can tell whether an action is good or bad if it makes sense for everyone to do it all the time. For example, is it okay to lie? No, because if everyone always lied, society would fall apart.

His logic is even more useful in the fat-loss and health field. We are trying to become slim and healthy for the rest of our lives. We do not want to lose body fat now only to gain it back later. So if a program isn't flexible enough for us to follow it forever, forget it.

Whatever we do to lose body fat, we have to keep on doing it or we will gain all the body fat back. It is like pushing the accelerator pedal to make your car go sixty miles per hour. As soon as you stop pushing it, you will slow down. Similarly, if you change the way you eat and exercise to burn body fat and then stop eating and exercising that way, you will quickly regain body fat. For instance, the *American Journal of Physiology* reported that as soon as rats stopped eating less, they gained weight twenty times faster than normal until they returned to at least their original weight.

Nobody wants to gain body fat twenty times faster than normal, so before trying any diet or exercise program, be a philosopher and ask yourself, "Can I do this forever?" If the answer is yes, do it. If the answer is no, skip it.

7

Calorie-Quality Factor 1: Satiety

A calorie is not a calorie when it comes to filling us up and keeping us full. Ever notice how a six-pack of beer makes people eat more pizza while five cans of tuna or thirty cups of broccoli—the same quantity of calories—would make them uncomfortably full? The capacity of calories to make us and keep us full is called Satiety. The fewer calories needed to fill us up and the longer those calories keep us full, the higher the Satiety value of the food. The first measure of assessing the SANEity of a food is its Satiety.

A study published in the *Annals of Internal Medicine* followed ten obese patients with type 2 diabetes for twenty-one days, and found that the people who ate as much high-Satiety protein and natural fat as they wanted, while avoiding low-Satiety starches and sweets, unconsciously avoided 1,000 low-quality calories per day.[68] These participants then reported feeling as satisfied as other people in the study who ate 1,000 more lower-Satiety calories.

Why is eating 1,000 fewer low-quality calories per day useful? Didn't we just show how harmful starvation is? Yes, but we're not talking starvation here. When we eat high-Satiety food, we take in more food and much more nutrition, but unintentionally become full faster, stay full longer, and therefore automatically avoid overeating. More food, more nutrition, more energy, and unconsciously avoiding excessive calories is entirely different from less food, less nutrition, feeling hungry, and being tired and cranky all day. The surplus of nutrition and satisfaction from high-satiety food saves us from the side effects of starvation.

The primary areas in our brain influenced by high-Satiety food are the lateral hypothalamus and ventromedial hypothalamus. They tell us when we feel satisfied from eating. Their "you are satisfied" signals that tell us to stop eating are dependent on three factors:

1. How much do the calories we are eating stretch our digestive organs?
2. How much do the calories we are eating affect short-term Satiety hormones?
3. How much do the calories we are eating stimulate long-term Satiety hormones?

We can eat more high-Satiety food by focusing on foods that contain high amounts of water, fiber, and protein.* How much any given food stretches our stomach and other digestive organs is mostly determined by the amount of water and fiber in it. More water and fiber means bigger food, more stretch, and getting fuller and staying fuller longer. That is why 200 calories of wet, fibrous celery is more filling than 200 calories of dry, fiber-free gummy bears. Calorie for calorie, celery is about thirty times the size of gummy bears, stretches our stomach and other digestive organs much more, and is therefore much more satisfying.

The amount of protein that food contains is also important. Harvard researchers have found that the amount of protein in food affects the other two factors that influence whether our brain is telling us we are hungry or full: short- and long-term Satiety hormones. More calories from protein mean more "full" hormonal signals being sent to our brain.

---

* Fiber: "Dietary fiber, also known as roughage or bulk, includes all parts of plant foods that your body cannot digest or absorb. Unlike other food components such as fats, proteins or carbohydrates—which your body breaks down and absorbs—fiber isn't digested by your body" (Mayo Clinic, "Dietary Fiber: Essential for a Healthy Diet," MayoClinic.com, www.mayoclinic.com/health/fiber/NU00033, accessed March 20, 2011). Taking up space in our digestive system until it "keeps us regular," fiber keeps us full for a long time.

These scientific findings have been repeated in numerous clinical trials:

In a University of Washington study, participants ate an unlimited quantity of calories while having the proportion of protein in their diet increased from 15 percent to 30 percent. They responded by unconsciously avoiding 441 excess calories per day without feeling hungry.[69]

In a University of Sussex study, participants ate either a high-protein or a low-protein meal. The high-protein people unconsciously ate 26 percent less than the low-protein people at their next meal without feeling hungry.[70]

In a University of Leeds study, participants ate the exact same weight of food, but one group ate a higher percent from protein. The higher-protein group unconsciously ate at least 19 percent fewer calories than the lower-protein group without feeling hungry.[71]

In a Karolinska Hospital study, participants ate more or less protein for lunch. The more-protein group got full on 12 percent fewer calories at dinner than the less-protein group.[72]

The science is clear: More water, fiber, and protein mean more Satiety. More Satiety means we are too full for set-point-raising low-quality food.

8

Calorie-Quality Factor 2: Aggression

Calories vary in how likely they are to be stored as body fat. When we eat, our digestive system acts a bit like a traffic cop who tells calories where to go. How Aggressively calories approach this traffic cop determines their chances of being stored as body fat.

The traffic cop directs calories to repair, fuel, or fatten us—in that order. The cop first makes sure we have enough resources to rebuild anything that has broken down. Next, the cop keeps us doing whatever we are doing. Last, the cop seeks to protect us from starving. As long as we have a calm and consistent flow of calories coming into our system, the cop does a great job directing them.

However, as with ordinary civil unruliness, our body does not do its best work when dealing with a bunch of Aggressive requests all at once. When calories approach the traffic cop Aggressively, the cop gets angry, throws its clipboard down, and locks up those calories in fat cells. Right after we eat a plate of pasta and a breadstick, a massive wave of starch starts screaming all at once and the traffic cop says, "Oh, really? To the fat cells . . . all of you!"

To keep calories from being locked up in our fat cells, we don't need to worry about eating less food. Our body is fine with a lot of food—it is the Aggressive food that annoys it. Five hundred calm calories creeping into the bloodstream over many hours are less likely to be stored as body fat than five hundred Aggressive calories rushing in all at once. Anytime the body has more calories available than it can deal with at one time, it stores them as body fat. That is why the *glycemic index* and *glycemic load* have become all the rage.* These handy measures of calories' Aggression are like the Most Wanted signs at the post office—they highlight the most dangerous Aggressive offenders.

To best understand calories' Aggression, glycemic index, and glycemic load, we first need to understand how our body fuels itself. Our body doesn't run on the food we eat—most often it runs on glucose, a sugar our body creates *from* the food we eat. That may seem like a meaningless distinction, but it is not.

Body-fat storage is not caused by eating a lot of food. Body-fat storage is triggered as a response to eating food that causes us to have more glucose in our bloodstream than we can use at one time. The more Aggressive calories are, the faster they increase the levels of glucose in our bloodstream. The faster calories increase our glucose levels, the more likely we are to have more glucose than the body can deal with at one time. That's when the traffic cop shuttles the excess into our fat cells.

The distinction between "a lot of food" and "a lot of glucose *right now*" is important. We can eat pounds and pounds of food and avoid pounds and pounds of body fat if the glucose the food generates does not exceed the glucose level our body can accommodate right then. That's the primary reason why the glycemic index, glycemic load, and low-glycemic diets like the South Beach Diet and the Atkins Diet work for so many people. These tools help people avoid excessive levels of blood glucose/blood sugar, a common trap that's easy for us to fall into, as our body needs surprisingly little glucose yet the normal Western diet is full of foods that spike blood sugar.

Researchers and authors Steve Phinney, MD, PhD, and Jeff Volek, PhD, RD, share a fascinating detail: our body has about *40 calories*

---

*Glycemic index: A measure of foods' Aggression. The higher a food's glycemic index, the more Aggressive it is.

Glycemic load: A measure that is similar to glycemic index but also considers quantity. The glycemic load measures a food's Aggression combined with the calories in a portion of it.

worth of glucose in circulation at any given time. "This means that when you digest . . . a cup of mashed potatoes or rice, most of the *200 calories* of glucose entering the bloodstream . . . has to be rapidly cleared to someplace else to keep blood sugar in the normal range."[73] That "someplace else" is generally our fat cells. So if we want to keep those calories out of our fat cells, we would be better off eating foods that are less Aggressive.

Fortunately, we don't need to worry about memorizing the glycemic index or glycemic load of foods because SANE eating prevents excess glucose from getting into our bloodstream. If we stick to increasing the amount of water-, fiber-, and protein-packed high-Satiety foods we are eating, we will automatically eat low-glycemic-index foods, ensure a low glycemic load, store less body fat, and lower our risk of coronary heart disease, diabetes, unhealthy cholesterol levels, and cardiovascular disease.*

---

* The fat in food is completely unAggressive. It does not increase the amount of glucose in the bloodstream at all. In fact, fat slows the release of glucose into the bloodstream. That is why foods containing fat are often less Aggressive than fat-free foods. That said, foods made up of nothing but fat—oils, butter, cream etc.—are not particularly SANE because they are not especially Satisfying, Nutritious, or in-Efficient. They are fine in moderation, but don't go crazy with them. We'll cover dietary fat in detail later.

Calorie-Quality Factor 3: Nutrition

Two hundred and fifty calories of Twinkies are not the same as 250 calories of broccoli. Calories are clearly different when it comes to discussing the Nutrition we need to burn body fat and be healthy. So what is nutritious? As with everything else, the key to Nutrition is *quality*—but all we are ever told about is quantity, the nutrition facts labels on food.

The information found on food labels tells us only half of what determines Nutrition quality: the quantity of nutrients in the food. But talking merely about the quantity of nutrients in food leads to a very fattening view of Nutrition. Consider the American Heart Association's endorsement logos on boxes of sugar-stuffed cereal because the cereal was "enriched." A high quantity of nutrients combined with low-quality calories is not nutritious. We know that ten doughnuts are not ten times as nutritious as one doughnut.

The other half of what determines Nutrition quality is the amount and characteristics of the calories we are getting along with the nutrients. We have to consider nutrients relative to calories.

Determining nutrition quality is simple. We take the nutrient quantity information provided on nutrition labels and divide it by the number of calories in a serving of the food. This provides the food's nutrition *per calorie*. Many nutrients per calorie—provided by nonstarchy vegetables, seafood, high-quality meats and dairy, low-fructose fruits, and nuts/seeds—means high nutrition quality. Few nutrients per calorie, provided by starches and sweets, means low nutrition quality.*

For example, here's how one cup of enriched wheat flour compares with one cup of spinach in terms of nutrient *quantity*. I've shaded the cell of the food with more of the given nutrient when we measure by the cup.

Nutrient *Quantity* of Enriched Wheat Flour versus Spinach
(Nutrients per Cup)

Nutrients (% DV)[†]	Enriched Wheat Flour	Spinach
Vitamin A	0%	56%
Vitamin C	0%	14%
Vitamin E	3%	3%
Vitamin K	1%	181%
Thiamin	74%	2%
Riboflavin	41%	3%
Niacin	52%	1%
Vitamin B_6	3%	3%
Folate	63%	15%
Calcium	2%	3%
Iron	34%	5%
Magnesium	9%	6%
Phosphorus	13%	1%
Potassium	4%	5%
Zinc	8%	1%

†DV: Recommended daily value based on a 2,000-calorie diet.

Looking at quantity, enriched wheat flour seems more nutritious than spinach in nutrients such as thiamin, niacin, folate, and iron. But

* Nonstarchy vegetables: The most SANE vegetables. Think of these as the vegetables you can eat raw and generally find in salads such as spinach, romaine lettuce, kale, any green leafy vegetable, broccoli, mushrooms, peppers, onions, zucchini, cauliflower, carrots, asparagus, etc. Basically anything other than corn, potatoes, turnips, yams, parsnips, radishes, etc. Corn, potatoes, yams, and other starchy foods are not SANE.

here's why that's misleading: One cup of enriched wheat flour contains 495 calories. One cup of spinach contains 7 calories. Looking at quality—nutrients *per calorie*—we see something much different—and more useful.

Nutrient *Quality* of Enriched Wheat Flour versus Spinach
(Nutrients per 250 Calories)

Nutrients (% DV)*	Enriched Wheat Flour	Spinach
Vitamin A	0%	2,000%
Vitamin C	0%	500%
Vitamin E	2%	107%
Vitamin K	1%	6,464%
Thiamin	37%	71%
Riboflavin	21%	107%
Niacin	26%	36%
Vitamin B_6	2%	107%
Folate	32%	536%
Calcium	1%	107%
Iron	17%	179%
Magnesium	5%	214%
Phosphorus	7%	36%
Potassium	2%	179%
Zinc	4%	36%

*DV: Recommended daily value based on a 2,000-calorie diet.

When we make a fair comparison—comparing 250 calories of enriched wheat flour against 250 calories of spinach, instead of comparing 495 calories of enriched wheat flour against 7 calories of spinach—we see that spinach is dramatically more nutritious than enriched wheat flour. Focusing on nutrition quality allows us to have a more accurate view of which foods are actually good for us.

Like Satiety and Aggression, a food's Nutrition depends on water, fiber, and protein. Water and fiber have no calories, and protein calories do not "count" as much as carbohydrate or fat calories (more on this in the next chapter). Since a food's nutrition quality is found by dividing the number of nutrients by the number of calories, more water, fiber, and protein reduce the relative number of calories in the food and thereby increase its nutrition quality.

Keeping water, fiber, and protein at the top of our mind in thinking about nutrition quality immediately gives us a dramatically different view of which foods are nutritious. Consider cereal, bread, or "healthy" whole-grain starches. They are all dry and contain little protein, so they are starting out zero for two. Fiber is their only hope.

The companies that sell starchy foods typically say we get a great deal of fiber from their whole-grain products, but is that actually true? The four grams of fiber in 250 calories of whole-grain cereal are 100 percent more fiber than the two grams of fiber in 250 calories of refined-grain cereal, but that is only comparing grains. We have to ask if grains are a good source of essential nutrients relative to more water- and protein-packed foods we could be eating. Sadly, whole grains are not good sources of essential nutrients relative to non-starches.

While whole grains are better than processed grains, one broken leg is also better than two—being better doesn't necessarily make something desirable. Look at the fiber *per calorie* in whole grains compared with more water- and protein-packed foods:

GRAMS OF FIBER IN 250 CALORIES

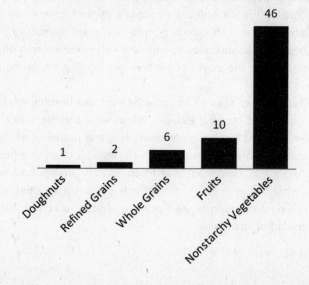

Whole grains do have six times more fiber than doughnuts, but nonstarchy vegetables have nearly fifty times more fiber. Whole-grain toast is better than a doughnut, but that is not saying much considering the other foods we could be eating. For example, if we eat 250 calories worth of nonstarchy vegetables, we will get about forty-six grams of fiber. To get the same amount of fiber from whole grains, we would have to eat nearly 2,000 calories worth of whole-grain bread. Eating whole-grain bread to get more fiber is like eating carrot cake to get more vegetables.

Starch is an excellent example of how careful we have to be when we consider the nutritive value of food. We could be eating all sorts of whole-grain starches thinking we are at the top of the nutrition mountain, while we are actually weighed down and sitting at the bottom. Few essential nutrients plus a lot of unSatisfying and Aggressive calories are not a winning combination.

Fortunately for us, we do not need to do all sorts of math with nutrition labels to maximize the nutrition quality of our diets. Researchers at Colorado State University did the math for us. They analyzed the nutrition quality of the most common foods and found that if we maximize the Satiety and minimize the Aggression of our diet—by eating more water-, fiber-, and protein-packed foods—we will get the most nutrition per calorie automatically. If you would like to calculate nutrition quality for yourself, the math is easy and informative. For instance, carefully check the foods people call "good sources of protein," such as beans, milk, and nuts. Are these foods good sources of protein per calorie? Divide the grams of protein in a serving by the number of calories.

Nutrition quality also affects whether we are burning body fat or slowing down and burning muscle. When we eat more water-, fiber-, and protein-packed food, we get more essential nutrients while avoiding overeating or overwhelming the body with glucose. Combine *more* nutrients with less overeating and fewer glucose spikes and we burn body fat without the negative side effects of starvation dieting. A surplus of essential nutrition is the opposite of starvation and our key to fat loss instead of frustration.

GRAMS OF PROTEIN IN A 250-CALORIE SERVING

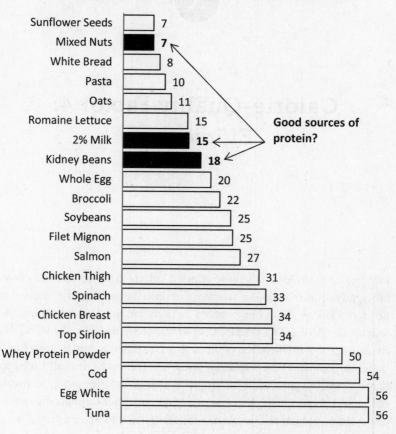

Sunflower Seeds	7
Mixed Nuts	7
White Bread	8
Pasta	10
Oats	11
Romaine Lettuce	15
2% Milk	15
Kidney Beans	18
Whole Egg	20
Broccoli	22
Soybeans	25
Filet Mignon	25
Salmon	27
Chicken Thigh	31
Spinach	33
Chicken Breast	34
Top Sirloin	34
Whey Protein Powder	50
Cod	54
Egg White	56
Tuna	56

Good sources of protein?

Calorie-Quality Factor 4: Efficiency

Last but far from least, a calorie is not a calorie when it comes to how Efficiently our metabolism converts it into body fat. The more inEfficient calories are at being stored as body fat, the better. Keeping the science of SANE eating simple, fiber and protein are entirely inEfficient. Explaining the inEfficiency of fiber is easy. Fiber is not digested and therefore can never be stored as body fat. The body tries and tries to digest fiber, but then after burning a bunch of calories trying to break down and absorb fiber, it gives up and passes fiber through the digestive system—which also explains why fiber helps to keep us regular.

Explaining the inEfficiency of protein is a bit more involved, but quite interesting. To start with let's talk about the calories we burn digesting food. It takes our body five to ten times more energy to digest protein than it does to digest fat or carbohydrate. In fact, about 30 percent of the calories we get from protein are burned in digesting it. Protein's inEfficiency doesn't stop there.

Even after we burn 30 percent of protein calories during initial digestion, protein cannot be directly stored as body fat. In contrast, a superhighway is busy shuttling glucose to our fat cells. So when we have excess protein lying around, it is sent to the liver to be converted into glucose. The process of converting protein into glucose is called gluconeogenesis (*gluco* = sugar, *neo* = new, *genesis* = creation). This process burns 33 percent of the remaining protein calories. Take the 70 percent of initial protein calories remaining after digestion and burn 33 percent of that during gluconeogenesis, and we are left with a measly 47 percent of the original protein calories.* What started off as, say, 300 calories of juicy protein is reduced to 140 calories of glucose in the bloodstream. Converting that newly formed glucose into body fat consumes 25 percent of the glucose calories. So when everything is said and done, only 35 percent of the initial calories we get from protein can be stored as body fat. You read that correctly. Over two-thirds of calories from protein are burned converting protein into a compound that can be stored as body fat. If we followed the same digestion process for starch, we would find that 211 of 300 starch calories can be stored as body fat. That means 70 percent of calories from starch can be stored as body fat. In other words, calories from starch are more than twice as Efficient at becoming body fat as calories from protein.

	Calories from Protein	Calories from Starch
Eaten	300	300
Digested	210	282
Converted into Glucose	140	282
Converted into Body Fat	105.5	211
105.5 × 2 = 211 **Calories from starch are twice as Efficient at being converted into body fat as calories from protein.**		

* The math here is a bit confusing, so let me explain how I've arrived at these numbers. Let's start with 100 calories of protein and convert it to amino acids; this process burns 30 percent of the calories, giving us 70 calories (or 70 percent of the original number). We then convert amino acids to glucose; this burns 33 percent of the 70 remaining calories, giving us about 47 calories (or 47 percent of the original 100). Finally we convert the glucose to body fat; this burns 25 percent of the remaining 47 calories, leaving us with only 35 calories (or 35 percent of the original 100). For the 300 calories given as an example in the text, we get: 70 percent of 300 = 210; then 210 − (210 × 0.33) = 210 − 69.3 = 140.7; then 140.7 − (140.7 × 0.25) = 140.7 − 35.2 = 105.7. Rounding, we get 105.5 as in the table, and that is about 35 percent of the original 300 calories.

This research doesn't suggest we should eat 100 percent protein. But it is suggesting that we can eat more and burn more by eating more protein-packed (and fiber-packed) food. And to keep things simple, the same techniques we are using to increase Satiety, decrease Aggression, and increase Nutrition also decrease the Efficiency of our calories.

HOW BODY FAT IS CREATED

With all this talk of calories being more or less Efficient at being stored as body fat, let's quickly cover how body fat gets created. The process of creating new body fat is called lipogenesis (*lipo* = fat and *genesis* = creation). And with genesis in mind: in the beginning there was food and food was classified by its dominant macronutrient.

Proteins	Fats	Carbohydrate
Seafood	Eggs	Everything Else*
Some meats	Tofu	
Egg whites	Oils	
Low-fat and low-sugar dairy	Nuts and seeds	
Low-sugar protein powders	Some meat	
	Full-fat dairy	

* Vegetables, fruit, most dairy, beans, and everything else are carbohydrates. They are not proteins or fats, so what else could they be?

As soon as our body is fed proteins, fats, or carbohydrates, it turns them into amino acids, fatty acids, or glucose, respectively. This first step is important because it provides another example of why a calorie is not a calorie. Once fat is converted to fatty acids, if there are more fatty acids around than we currently need, all of them are sent off to be stored as body fat. The glucose we get from carbohydrates does not work that way. Glucose cannot be stored as body fat without the hormone insulin. And then there are the inEfficient amino acids from protein. Amino acids must first be converted into glucose. Once they become glucose, they need insulin or they cannot be stored as body fat.

Now let's assume the hormone insulin is making its rounds and we have excess glucose on its way to fat cells. At that point, glucose is converted into fatty acids and we are one step away from new body fat. During the last step in the process, all those fatty acids combine

FROM FOOD TO BODY FAT

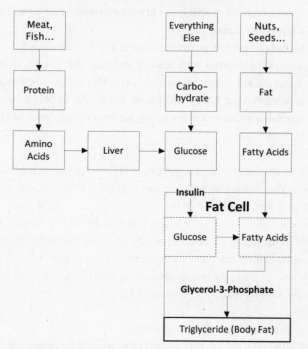

with a glycerol molecule to form triglyceride—body fat. This is called esterification and it is not possible without a substance called glycerol-3-phosphate.

Why am I telling you about how our bodies create fat? Because once you understand the science, there are three useful takeaways:

1. Not all calories are the same, considering that protein is five calorie-burning steps away from body fat—convert into amino acids, convert to glucose, meet up with insulin, transform to fatty acids, and hook up with glycerol-3-phosphate—while fat is only two calorie-burning steps away: convert into fatty acids and hook up with glycerol-3-phosphate.

2. It is impossible to store glucose as body fat without enough insulin. The more Aggressive a calorie is, the more insulin it triggers the pancreas to release. This can overwork the system and lead to cells becoming insulin resistant. Eventually, if too much insulin is triggered too often,

the pancreas can wear out, resulting in type 2 diabetes (we'll cover this in more detail later). That is one of the major reasons we want to avoid Aggressive calories.

3. No body fat gets stored without glycerol-3-phosphate. We get the most glycerol-3-phosphate from inSANE starches and sweets. Carbohydrates are not all bad—nonstarchy vegetables are carbohydrates and they are the most SANE foods around. But inSANE carbohydrates from starches and sweets fuel overeating, set-point dysregulation, and body-fat formation.

Put this all together and it becomes clear why eating as many SANE calories as you want will keep you at a healthy body weight long term, while eating less does not. When people eat less, their body believes they are still overeating, since their metabolism slows down. Additionally, they have plenty of insulin and glycerol-3-phosphate thanks to the inSANE low-quality starches and sweets they continue eating. Overeating plus insulin and glycerol-3-phosphate means new body fat.

On the other hand, when we go SANE:

We avoid overeating thanks to high-Satiety.
Calories are released into our bloodstream slowly and they trigger little insulin thanks to low Aggression.
Our bodies benefit from a number of essential nutrients thanks to high-Nutrition.
We burn a lot of calories during digestion thanks to low-Efficiency.

Eating all this SANE food makes us too full for inSANE starches and sweets. By avoiding starches and sweets, we do not have a surplus of calories to store and we don't have enough insulin or glycerol-3-phosphate to fuel excess body fat formation. Free from the need or ability to store body fat, we eat more food and slim down.

Before we dig deeper into the day-to-day details of eating more—but smarter—there is one more calorie myth we must free ourselves from: calories are everything, so moderation is all that matters.

How to Eat SANE as a Vegetarian: Cristina's Story

A SANE lifestyle is compatible with plant-based, paleo, primal, low-carb, organic, local, vegetarian, kosher, halal, or virtually any other lifestyle. It's about eating Satisfying, unAggressive, Nutritious, and inEfficient food. If you would like to add other criteria, that's no problem.

For example, Cristina is a vegetarian who went SANE by dramatically increasing her intake of nonstarchy vegetables, enjoying plant-based protein, and savoring whole-food fats such as nuts and seeds.

How did SANEitizing her vegetarian lifestyle work out for Cristina? In her words:

> I have plenty to eat. I am not starving. On the contrary, I am well-nourished and satisfied and feel great all the time. Three months of eating like this has gotten me off a diabetes medication and reduced my HbA1C from 8.3 to 5.7, rendering me diabetes-free. I also was on cholesterol medication, but after I "SANEitized" my eating, my cholesterol went from 220 to 103, and I was taken off that medication as well.
>
> My husband, who is not a vegetarian but humors me and eats what I eat inside the house and orders lean meats when we go out, has lost 32 pounds, resolved his sleep apnea, and stopped having migraines. We both stopped having heartburn, which for me was a daily and painful occurrence—no doubt, starch and sugar related. And to top it off, I have lost 45 pounds in three months!
>
> There's just one more thing: After five years of trying, I finally got pregnant! I can't tell you how excited my husband and I are. You better believe we'll be SANE for life now.

SANEity isn't about "you must do this" and "you can never do that." It is about using simple science instead of complex myths to live better—whatever your lifestyle.

The Myth of Moderation

The "classical theory" that fat is deposited in the adipose tissue [body fat] only when given in excess of the caloric requirement is finally disproved.

—Ernst Wertheimer, in *Physiological Reviews*[74]

The final myth complicating our lives and destroying our health is the idea that calories are the most important consideration in our food choices, so we can eat anything we'd like as long as we're careful to analyze food labels for serving sizes and calories. So here is our third Calorie Myth:

Calorie Myth #3: All Foods Are Fine in Moderation

Most diets suggest that we can eat whatever we want and be fine as long as we monitor our portion sizes and don't eat too many calories. But as we've discussed, calories are not all that matter. What comes along with calories can disrupt our fundamental biology for generations. So why do we hear so much about calories and eating "everything" in moderation? One reason is that many of the institutions perpetuating this myth are funded by companies that produce processed foods. These institutions can keep their corporate benefactors happy and appear reasonable by preaching a message of moderation. (*The "foods" aren't bad—your willpower is! It's your "personal responsibility" to resist them!*) Now anyone can sell anything and everyone is happy—except for the consumers whose biology is being broken.

WHY HORMONES MATTER MORE THAN MODERATION

When we are told to focus on calories and moderation instead of food and biology, "healthy" quickly becomes a highly relative term. For example, a popular fast food chain celebrates the health benefits of its offerings that contain less than 400 calories. Never mind the high-fructose corn syrup, refined flour, trans fats, and pink slime in these edible products we collectively refer to as "food," they're low calorie and therefore "smart" choices.

We know this is absurd. We know that the nutritional and hormonal impact of calories matters immensely. But we can see why the calorie craze is perpetuated. Want to sell anything and call it healthy? Convince people calories are all that matter. Then mix together the cheapest and most shelf-stable ingredients you can find and call it edible. Finally, shrink the serving size until you can call it low calorie and therefore "healthy." One-hundred-calorie snack packs for everyone!

Misguided recommendations around moderation are not new. Just a few decades ago we were given a message of smoking in moderation, but then the science linking smoking to addiction and disease became clear. The link between inSANE foods addiction and disease is now clear. As Yale University's Kelly Brownell puts it, "By 1964, there was sufficient scientific evidence . . . [but] many years passed and many millions died before decisive action was taken to [turn the tide against smoking]. . . . Repeating this history with food and obesity would be tragic."[75]

Will a single soda or candy bar every once in a while kill us? Of course not. But neither will a single cigarette every once in a while. The question is what we should be *recommending*. The message of moderation and calories is rooted in money, not science. Accurate recommendation would revolve around food quality and hormones, not calorie count and moderation.

THE SIMPLE SCIENCE OF HORMONES

At the risk of being a little gruesome (I'd suggest putting down your fork if you're reading this book while eating a SANE meal), let's look at one way scientists discovered the important relationship between hormones and health: through a procedure known as parabiosis. Parabiosis occurs when researchers cut two live animals open and then

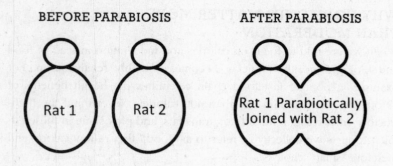

BEFORE PARABIOSIS   **AFTER PARABIOSIS**

Rat 1   Rat 2   Rat 1 Parabiotically Joined with Rat 2

join them so they share the same blood supply and hormones. In other words, researchers create conjoined twins.

Why would researchers create a Franken-rat with one set of hormones but twice as much of everything else? Because it allows them to investigate the impact of hormones on human health. For example, when researchers join an obese rat to a lean rat, the lean rat gets leaner regardless of the quantity of calories it eats. How is that possible? Think back to how the set-point works.[76]

The obese rat is producing a massive amount of body-fat-burning hormones in an effort to get itself back to a normal level of body fat. But because the obese rat is clogged and cannot respond to the body-fat-burning hormones effectively, it stays heavy. However, the lean rat is not clogged. The lean and clog-free rat *is* able to respond to all those body-fat-burning hormones.

Lots of body-fat-burning hormones + the ability to respond to them = burning body fat despite eating the same quantity of calories.

Similarly, when researchers stitch a normal rat and a starved rat together, the starved rat's body-fat-storing hormones make the normal rat get fatter without eating any more calories. The starved rat is producing body-fat-storing hormones in an effort to get back to its set-point. These body-fat-storing hormones enter the normal rat, and it does exactly what the hormones tell it to do: the normal rat stores body fat without eating any more or exercising any less.

Besides the horror of joining living animals together, these studies powerfully demonstrate how any message regarding eating or exercise that doesn't involve hormones is at best incomplete. And that is only the tip of the investigative iceberg.

Researchers at the Veterans Affairs Palo Alto Health Care System genetically altered mice so they would no longer have a primary enzyme responsible for storing body fat (hormone-sensitive lipase). These mice ate
more and gained 70 percent less than normal mice. In the researchers'
words, completely independently of calories, altering mice's hormones
caused "a drastic reduction in lipogenesis [body fat creation]."[77]

Researchers at the University of Basel genetically altered mice's hormone
levels so that the mice stayed lean, "in spite of reduced physical activity," and were "unaffected [by] caloric intake."[78]

Peter Havel from the University of California tells us that "mice which are
unable to produce ASP [a hormone involved in the formation of body fat]
consume 30 percent more food than wild-type mice, yet have reduced
adipose [body fat] mass and are resistant to weight gain."[79]

These and hundreds of other experiments show that hormones
are the key to our set-point and therefore long-term weight gain or
loss. The journal *Neuroscience & Biobehavioral Reviews* captures the
importance of healing our hormones before we are permanently free
of body fat: "humans that become obese gain weight because they are
no longer able to lose weight."[80] We gain weight because our metabolic
system is hormonally broken. Starving a broken system will never fix
it; there's a good chance it will make it worse. We fix the problem by
understanding and healing our hormones.

HOW HORMONES INFLUENCE OUR SET-POINT

Our digestive system, muscle tissue, and fat tissue are constantly communicating with our nervous system and brain via hormones. They
are talking about how much fuel they think we need to keep us at our
set-point. If they think we are at risk of rising above our set-point, they
automatically decrease our calories in and increase our calories out,
and vice versa.

When we eat SANE high-quality calories, this conversation goes
well. Higher-quality calories trigger body-fat-burning hormones. The
right amount of hormones are used and the right message is communi-
cated: "Burn body fat."

However, when we eat inSANE low-quality calories, communication
breaks down. Our body doesn't have a good idea of how much fuel we

need, hormones become "dysregulated,"[81] and our body demands more food, since it does not know what is going on and errs on the side of not starving. Thanks to this communication breakdown, we overeat, become hormonally clogged, and gain weight. You can count calories all day and will not set yourself up for *long-term* fat loss if you are eating low-quality calories that trigger excess body-fat-storing hormones such as insulin.

Known in scientific circles as the most important hormonal factor influencing body fat creation, insulin is activated only when we need to get fuel into our cells. Our body "hears" insulin in the bloodstream "communicating" that we have energy on its way to our cells and therefore do not need to use any stored energy—i.e., burn body fat. So the hormone insulin—not the calories we ate—blocks the burning of body fat.

Calories from inSANE starch and sweets trigger the release of ridiculous amounts of insulin. All that insulin gets those calories into our cells, but then we still have insulin left over in our bloodstream. That excess insulin clogs us up and removes our ability to burn body fat no matter how much time we spend on the treadmill.

Things go from bad to worse if we keep this up for too long. Not only does all the excess insulin destroy our ability to burn body fat, it also makes our body resistant to insulin (meaning that our pancreas has to produce more insulin to do the same job). To quickly understand how this works, think about this analogy: becoming resistant to the effects of insulin is like becoming resistant to the effects of alcohol. When people drink alcohol in moderation, everything is fine. It takes relatively little alcohol to generate the desired effect, so people don't drink too much of it. However, if people drink too much alcohol, they become resistant to alcohol's effects and then they have to drink more to get a buzz. This volume of alcohol eventually destroys their liver and makes them sick.

Similarly, when people eat mostly SANE foods, everything is fine. It takes just a little insulin to get energy into cells, so the body doesn't produce too much of it. If our insulin levels remain low, we don't gain weight—even when we eat large amounts of food. Instead of being stored as fat, extra blood-sugar-increasing calories are burned off or eventually exit the body as waste. But if people eat a significant amount

WHERE THE AVERAGE AMERICAN GETS CALORIES

**Insulin-spiking starch and sweeteners
make up 43 percent of what we eat.**

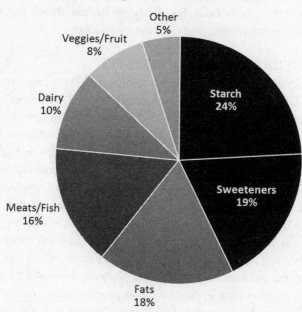

Other
5%

Veggies/Fruit
8%

Dairy
10%

Starch
24%

Meats/Fish
16%

Sweeteners
19%

Fats
18%

of starch and sweets, their bodies become resistant to insulin's effects. Then their bodies have to produce more insulin to get energy into cells. This volume of insulin eventually destroys their pancreas and makes them sick. Insulin resistance is becoming an epidemic in our country. At least one in four Americans is insulin resistant. All this excess insulin forms the backbone of our clog and causes our set-point to creep up. It also increases the rate at which we store body fat because excess insulin preferentially puts calories into our fat tissue. No matter how resistant other tissues become to insulin, our fat tissue is always receptive. While that is technically good because it keeps insulin resistance from killing us (it prevents toxically high levels of blood sugar), it can prevent us from losing weight. We end up with more body fat and no ability to burn it.

Once most of the calories we eat are being stored in fat cells because insulin cannot get them into other cells, *internal starvation* has set in. We eat plenty of food but starve on the inside because insulin cannot effectively get that energy into any cells other than our fat cells. With excess insulin shuttling most calories into fat tissue and eliminating our ability to burn body fat, the body has no choice but to slow down, burn muscle tissue, and demand more food.

THE ACTUAL CAUSE OF OBESITY

Meet Terri. She is internally starving and needs 500 calories of energy. Terri is also a yo-yo dieter and has already slowed down her metabolism and burned as much muscle as she can. Needing some calories, Terri eats 500 calories. Instead of those 500 calories getting into the organs needing it, only 250 make it in while the other 250 are ignored—thanks to insulin resistance—and stored as new body fat. Terri still needs 250 calories. She cannot slow down anymore. She cannot burn any more muscle. And thanks to all the excess insulin floating around, she does not have the ability to burn body fat. What is her only option? Overeat. Eat 250 extra calories. So Terri snacks on 250 extra calories to keep her cells from starving. But now only some of the 250 calories make it to the cells needing them while the rest are stored as body fat. Again, she must overeat even more. This process of overeating to keep a clogged body fueled repeats itself until Terri eats 1,000 calories to meet her need for 500 calories. Terri's body is leaking calories into her fat cells and has to compensate by taking in extra calories. Continue this "overeat to compensate for the clog" cycle day after day and Terri gains body fat. On the surface it seems that she is gaining body fat because she is eating too many calories. But Terri's high consumption of calories is not the *cause* of her weight gain. It is a *symptom* of the hormonal clog caused by inSANE low-quality calories.

Obesity is not caused by eating too many calories and it is not cured by eating fewer calories. Overeating is not the cause of obesity, says Hilde Bruch at Baylor University. "It is a symptom of an underlying disturbance. . . . The changes in weight regulation and fat storage are the essential disturbances."[82]

Problems are not solved by treating symptoms. That is why the Calorie Myths fail more than 95 percent of the time. Basing your diet on calorie count is like taking a medication that treats the symptoms of an

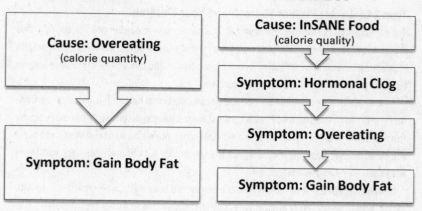

illness, but doesn't cure the underlying cause. We can monitor our bodies all we want by tracking calories in versus calories out, but if we're not eating foods that fuel our biological processes and help to regulate our hormones, we're not curing our bodies.

Now that we've walked through each of the Calorie Myths, I want to spend a little time talking about how these myths were created in the first place. Why haven't you heard about this science until now? Sadly, financial motivation is part of the answer. More money can be made off sick, overweight, and unhappy people than off healthy, fit, and happy people. The bigger we are, the bigger the profits of the $3.1 trillion food, $150 billion fitness, and $500 billion pharmaceutical industries.

Big food, big fitness, and big pharma want us to stay slim the way big tobacco wants us to stop smoking. You can't believe everything you hear. Especially if it is coming from a person or organization whose profits depend on your continued weight and health struggles. As SUNY professor Jeffrey M. Friedman explains, "Why has the scientific evidence from long-standing obesity research not found its way into the minds of the public . . . ? Perhaps it is because these views are shaped by a constant barrage of advertisements from the diet industry which has a multi-billion dollar interest in promoting the view that weight can be controlled through volition [willpower] alone."[83]

Type 2 Diabetes: Protect Yourself and Your Children

Type 2 diabetes is like running water into a hormonally clogged sink for so long that water overflows all over the place and the faucet breaks down. Once so much insulin is produced that it is overflowing in our bloodstream and our ability to produce insulin has broken down, we develop type 2 diabetes.

This buildup and breakdown cause potentially lethal havoc in the body. The Centers for Disease Control and Prevention estimates people diagnosed with diabetes by the age of forty die twelve years sooner if they are male and fourteen years sooner if they are female. We can only imagine the years lost for children who are saturated with starches and sweets.

Type 2 diabetes is terrible. What is even worse is its disturbing growth. In the late 1800s, one in every 4,000 people was diabetic; today one in every four people is diabetic or prediabetic. That is a 100,000 percent increase in one century, and researchers estimate that we are on our way to a third of men and nearly a half of women in the United States becoming type 2 diabetic. The worst is yet to come.

Exposure to a diabetic and hormonally clogged environment in utero will impair a baby's ability to regulate the set-point-related hormones insulin and leptin, while permanently adding fat cells to his or her body and increasing the child's vulnerability to obesity, diabetes, and heart disease over the course of a lifetime. These findings are most compellingly demonstrated in studies in which researchers look at siblings of whom one was born before the mother became insulin resistant or diabetic and the other was born after (this setup holds genetics constant and helps researchers to limit the variables). Related studies in animals are equally scary. When pregnant animals are fed inSANE food, the genetic expression of their offspring is altered and causes the offspring to crave starches and sweets more than their parents do.

We are faced with the first generation with a lower life expectancy than their parents. About one in three American children is overweight or obese, and more than 40 million children *under the age of five* are overweight thanks in part to their exposure to hormonal havoc, elevated set-points, and inSANE cravings before they were even born. As University of Colorado's associate dean for faculty, Dana Dabelea, MD, PhD, puts it, "The effects of maternal diabetes . . . may be viewed as a vicious cycle. Children whose mothers had diabetes during pregnancy are at increased risk of becoming obese and developing diabetes at young ages. Many of these female offspring already have diabetes or abnormal glucose tolerance by the time they reach their childbearing years, thereby perpetuating the cycle."[84]

As alarming as this picture is, we still have plenty to be hopeful about. Remember Cristina's story? A series of more encouraging studies show that the vast majority of type 2 diabetics can reduce or completely eliminate their need for medication by going SANE, while significantly reversing insulin resistance via smarter exercise.

Where the Calorie Myths Came From

One way to clear up all the calorie confusion is to start at the beginning and look at the history of eating using a scale of one day. Say 12:00 a.m. was the dawn of our first ancestors and right now it's one second before midnight. Up until 11:57 p.m. our ancestors stayed healthy and fit, eating only what could be found directly in nature—vegetables, seafood, meat, eggs, fruits, nuts, and seeds. At 11:57 p.m. people started farming, became "civilized," and began eating starch and a small amount of sweets. Two seconds ago, people started eating processed starches and sweets. Only right now—one second before midnight—did people start getting most of their calories from genetically modified and highly manufactured starch- and sweetener-based edible products.

That means the diet recommended by the government's *Dietary Guidelines* was not possible—forget about healthy or slimming—for 99.8 percent of our history. Our ancestors did not hunt or gather pasta, rice, cereal, or bread. They did not eat whole grains. They ate no grains. They did not cut back on added sweeteners. They did not know what added sweeteners were. Emory University anthropologist S. Boyd Eaton, MD, tells us, "During the late Paleolithic [the vast majority of human history], the great majority of carbohydrates was derived from vegetables and fruit, very little from cereal grains and none from refined flours."[85]

This idea is interesting to think about when it comes to our health.

Obesity, diabetes, and heart disease are called "diseases of civilization." They did not become issues until agriculture enabled production of starches and sweets about twelve thousand years ago. They did not reach epidemic status until starches and sweets became highly processed, were genetically modified, and made up most of our diet. Colorado State University researchers found that a whopping 72 percent of what we eat today was not eaten for at least 99.8 percent of our evolutionary history.[86]*

How Much of Today's Typical Diet Is Not Natural?

Food	% Calories
Starches	**24%**
Whole Grains	4%
Refined Grains	20%
Added Sweeteners	**19%**
Sucrose	8%
High-Fructose Corn Syrup	8%
Glucose	3%
Refined Oils	**18%**
Salad, Cooking Oils	9%
Shortening	7%
Margarine	2%
Alcohol	**1%**
Dairy	**11%**
Milk	4%
Cheese	3%
Butter	1%
Other	3%
Total	**72%**

The diet we evolved to eat has been flipped on its head. Is it any wonder our health and fitness have been flipped on their heads as

* When I use the term "evolution" please feel free to read "human history" if that better fits within your lifestyle. If you prefer to read "human history," please also read "99.8 percent" as "95 percent" as human history is a shorter period of time than evolutionary history.

well? Over 70 percent of our diet is made up of unnatural food. Over 70 percent of us have unhealthy and inflated waistlines. Coincidence or common sense?

Of course, some people might object: "Back then, people didn't live as long as we do now." That is an excellent point. I felt the same way until I discovered research that reveals three facts about hunter-gatherers:

1. They are few and far between today, but hunter-gatherer tribes are still around, and scientists have studied them intensively. The studies show that they are free from obesity, diabetes, and heart disease.

2. While their *average* age of death is lower than ours, many ancient hunter-gatherers lived beyond the age of sixty. Back to Dr. S. Boyd Eaton: "Occasionally one hears the claim that primitive people all died too young to get degenerative diseases. This claim is simply false— many lived well into and through the age of vulnerability for such disorders, yet didn't get them." [87]

3. Let's take old age out of the equation entirely. Obese and type 2 diabetic "civilized" children are running around all over the place. The children of hunter-gatherers were free of obesity and diabetes.

It's not a coincidence that the decline in the quality of our food has coincided with the decline in the quality of our health. We are not designed to digest the majority of foods we're being told to eat. Walter Willett, chair of the Harvard School of Public Health, states unequivocally, "The USDA Pyramid is wrong. It was built on shaky scientific ground . . . [and] has been steadily eroded by new research from all parts of the globe. . . . At best, [it] offers wishy-washy, scientifically unfounded advice." [88] The *Journal of the American College of Cardiovascular Exerciselogy* makes this connection: "The low-fat-high-carbohydrate diet, promulgated vigorously by the . . . food pyramid, may well have played an unintended role in the current epidemics of obesity . . . diabetes, and metabolic syndromes." [89] Michael F. Jacobson, the cofounder of the Center for Science in the Public Interest, offers a blunt assessment: "Good advice about nutrition conflicts with the interests of many big industries, each of which has more lobbying power than all the public-interest groups combined." [90]

THE SOURCE OF OUR WEIGHT PROBLEMS

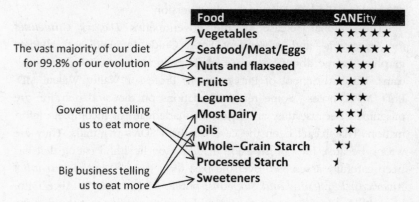

Food	SANEity
Vegetables	★ ★ ★ ★ ★
Seafood/Meat/Eggs	★ ★ ★ ★ ★
Nuts and flaxseed	★ ★ ★ ★⌐
Fruits	★ ★ ★
Legumes	★ ★ ★
Most Dairy	★ ★ ⌐
Oils	★ ★
Whole-Grain Starch	★ ⌐
Processed Starch	⌐
Sweeteners	

The vast majority of our diet for 99.8% of our evolution

Government telling us to eat more

Big business telling us to eat more

Decades of advanced dietary research have taken place alongside spiking obesity and disease rates. This research recommends a diet much different from any version of the government's *Dietary Guidelines*. For example, Marion Nestle, PhD, MD, professor of nutrition, food studies, and public health at New York University, notes how the scientific community has long criticized the USDA's Food Guide Pyramid's failure to recognize that sugar and starch are biochemically equivalent within the body. Starch has the same impact on our body as sugar, says Donald Layman, PhD, professor of nutrition at the University of Illinois. "All starches from all of the grains are simply a long chain of simple sugars connected together. The term complex carbohydrate just means a long chain of sugars. As soon as a food is digested and absorbed, the body does not know the difference between a simple sugar and a whole grain."[91]

Why don't the government's guidelines reflect this research? Why is a food that is "biochemically equivalent" to sugar *recommended* in mass quantities?[92]

A great deal of money is being made from our nutritional confusion. The history of the USDA guidelines and graphics is nothing short of shocking.

POLITICIANS PLAYING PHYSICIANS

Detailing the disturbing history of the government's role in our diet would take an entire book. If you would like to find out the whole story, you can read an excellent book called *Good Calories, Bad Calories* by Gary Taubes. Here is the short version.

The original release of the government's *Dietary Guidelines for Americans*—and subsequent Food Guide Pyramid and MyPlate graphics—came about because certain politicians were playing physicians. Harvard School of Public Health Professor Walter Willett, MD, PhD, MPH, notes: "Some recommendations on diet and nutrition are misguided because they are based on inadequate or incomplete information. That hasn't been the case for the USDA's pyramids. They are wrong because they brush aside evidence on healthful eating that has been carefully assembled over the past forty years."[93] In the *Journal of American Physicians and Surgeons*, public health scientist Alice Ottoboni, PhD, adds: "There is considerable concern today that the diet the Pyramid illustrates is responsible for the current epidemic of cardiovascular disease. The concurrent epidemics of obesity and type-2 diabetes are unintended consequences that can also be attributed to this diet."[94]

How did the government come up with these dietary guidelines? In 1980, when the guidelines were first introduced, scientists did not have a good understanding of what would happen if most people adopted these guidelines. The dietary guidelines and graphics were not drawn up by nutrition scholars. They were derived from a political document released in 1976 called *Dietary Goals for the United States.** *Dietary Goals* was designed by the Senate Select Committee on Nutrition and Human Needs to do two things. The first was to increase carbohydrate consumption to account for 55 percent to 60 percent of calorie intake. The second was to reduce overall fat consumption from 40 percent to about 30 percent of calorie intake.

These goals and the rest of the document are more speculative than scientific. Dr. Stewart Truswell, professor in the School of Molecular Bioscience at the University of Sydney, tells us, "The first edition of *Dietary Goals* . . . took nutritionists by surprise. . . . [It] was written by a group of politically interested activists with small knowledge of

* First there was *Dietary Goals* (1976), then came the *Dietary Guidelines* (1980), the Food Guide Pyramid (1992), MyPyramid (2005), and finally MyPlate (2011). Additionally, since the release of the original *Dietary Guidelines*, the government has rereleased the same basic guidance every five years.

nutrition. . . . The collected objections can be summarized very briefly: Too soon, more research needed, relationships not proved; politically motivated."[95] Even the American Medical Association was worried when *Dietary Goals* was released, lamenting the potentially harmful effects of such a radical long-term dietary change. Scientists at the University of Wisconsin–Madison called the goals report "not scientifically sound," referring to it as "a political and moralistic document."[96]

Perhaps the most telling objection came from the president of the National Academy of Sciences in his testimony to the Senate in regard to *Dietary Goals:* "What right has the federal government to propose that the American people conduct a vast nutritional experiment, with themselves as subjects, on the strength of so very little evidence that it will do them any good?"[97]

But although *Dietary Goals* was unproved and controversial among the scientific community, the government declared it "the truth" on these grounds: "We [the government] live in the present and cannot afford to await the ultimate proof before correcting trends we believe to be detrimental."[98] With that uneducated guess, a low-fat, low-protein, high-starch diet was declared "healthy." Sadly, the results have been anything but.

To understand why the Senate Nutrition Committee gave us these dietary goals in the first place, we have to go back a few more decades. One man single-handedly convinced the country that natural foods are deadly.

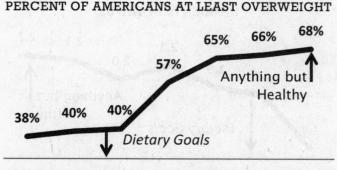

PERCENT OF AMERICANS AT LEAST OVERWEIGHT

38%   40%   40%   57%   65%   66%   68%

Anything but Healthy

Dietary Goals

'60–'62   '71–'74   '76–'80   '88–'94   '99–'02   '03–'04   '07–'08

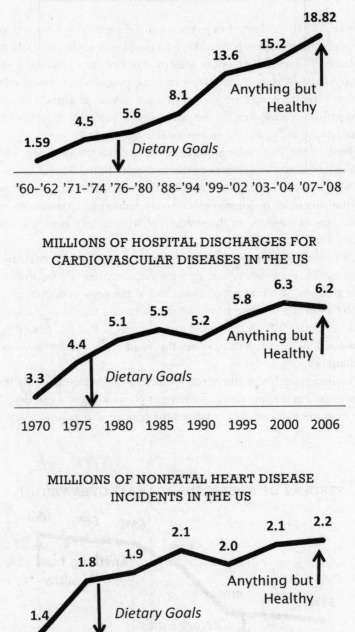

MILLIONS OF AMERICANS WITH DIABETES

18.82

15.2

13.6

8.1

5.6

4.5

1.59

Dietary Goals

Anything but
Healthy

'60–'62 '71–'74 '76–'80 '88–'94 '99–'02 '03–'04 '07–'08

MILLIONS OF HOSPITAL DISCHARGES FOR
CARDIOVASCULAR DISEASES IN THE US

6.3

6.2

5.8

5.5

5.2

5.1

4.4

3.3

Dietary Goals

Anything but
Healthy

1970 1975 1980 1985 1990 1995 2000 2006

MILLIONS OF NONFATAL HEART DISEASE
INCIDENTS IN THE US

2.1

2.1

2.2

2.0

1.9

1.8

1.4

Dietary Goals

Anything but
Healthy

1970 1975 1980 1985 1990 1995 2000

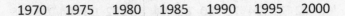

FAT FICTION

In the 1950s Ancel Keys examined diet and heart disease trends in twenty-two countries. He was apparently more interested in headlines than science because he then published a study that included data from only the *six* countries that showed a frightening link between dietary fat and heart disease. Keys garnered a massive amount of press and then went on tour armed with the message that eating fat is deadly.

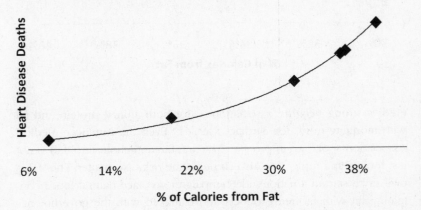

HEART DISEASE DEATHS PER 1,000 MEN

Japan, Italy, England, Australia, Canada, and the United States

Heart Disease Deaths

6%   14%   22%   30%   38%

% of Calories from Fat

Here are the facts: When the data from *all twenty-two* countries in Keys's study are examined, they show *no* relationship between dietary-fat intake and heart disease deaths. Keys selectively picked data and designed a headline-worthy conclusion. In the words of a fellow researcher, "No information is given by Keys on how or why the six countries were selected."[99] Further exposing the randomness of Keys's methods, those same researchers revealed that by selectively choosing six different countries from Keys's data, they could create a graph suggesting that eating *more* fat *decreases* the risk of dying from heart disease.

Finally, looking at Keys's data a few years later, they concluded, "The examination of *all* available basic data . . . show[s] that the association [between fat and heart disease] lacks validity."[100] They also discov-

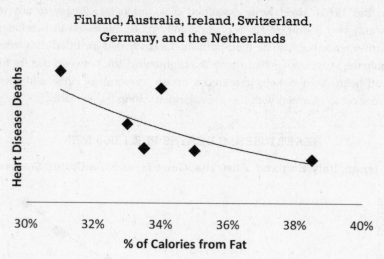

HEART DISEASE DEATHS PER 1,000 MEN

Finland, Australia, Ireland, Switzerland, Germany, and the Netherlands

ered "a strong *negative* association . . . for both animal protein and fat with mortality from non-cardiac diseases." Even the American Medical Association spoke up in protest: "The anti-fat, anti-cholesterol fad is not just foolish and futile . . . it also carries some risk." No matter. The "fat is evil" myth started a nationwide campaign to replace natural foods containing fat with fat-free products and climaxed with the government's *Dietary Guidelines*, Food Guide Pyramid, MyPyramid, and MyPlate diets. Those diets are high in starch because starch is low in fat. Unfortunately, over a billion dollars' worth of studies have failed to prove that the government's guidelines are good for anything other than profits.

Harvard Medical School's position on the government's eating guidelines is unambiguous: "Few public health messages are as powerful and as persistent as this one: Fat is bad. . . . The average American has substantially reduced the percentage of calories that she or he gets from fat over the past three decades. . . . But we are not any healthier for all of this effort. In fact, we are worse off for it."[101] Numerous studies have have been unable to find a link between dietary fat and heart disease.

When Patty W. Siri-Tarino, PhD, of the Children's Hospital & Research Center in Oakland, examined twenty-one studies that included a total of 347,747 people, he found, "There is *no* significant evidence for concluding that dietary saturated fat is associated with an increased risk of heart disease or cardiovascular disease."[102] The National Heart, Lung, and Blood Institute funded an enormous trial designed to link the consumption of foods containing fat to heart disease. The $115 million Multiple Risk Factor Intervention Trial took 12,866 men with high cholesterol, split them into two groups, and fed one group the government guidelines' diet for seven years with the hope of lowering the incidence of heart disease. The government's diet resulted in a 7.1 percent *increase* in heart disease deaths.[103]

The Women's Health Initiative of the National Institutes of Health completed a $700 million study to test the fat hypothesis. A whopping 48,835 women ate their normal diet or the government diet for about eight years. At the end of the study, the regular- and government-diet women weighed the same and no differences were found in their health. The researchers concluded, "Dietary intervention that reduced total fat intake did *not* significantly reduce the risk of coronary heart disease, stroke, or cardiovascular disease."[104] As reported in the study: "[This] trial is the largest long-term randomized trial of a dietary intervention ever conducted to our knowledge, and it achieved an 8.2 percent reduction . . . in total fat intake. . . . *No* significant effects on incidence of coronary heart disease or stroke were observed." On February 8, 2006, the *New York Times* ran the headline: LOW-FAT DIET DOES *NOT* CUT HEALTH RISKS, STUDY FINDS.

A massive study named MONICA involved 113 groups of scientists and doctors in twenty-seven countries studying everything they thought could contribute to heart disease. They found little if any association between the average cholesterol level and heart-related mortality. In the Western Electric Study—known in academic circles as one of "the most informative prospective studies to date"—researchers concluded, "Although the focus of dietary recommendations is usually a reduction of saturated fat intake, *no* relation between saturated fat intake and risk of coronary heart disease was observed [in their study]."[105]

The government was trying to help with the guidelines but, sadly, it failed. Harvard Medical School Professor of Medicine Frank Hu, MD, MPH, PhD, tells us, "It is now increasingly recognized that the low-fat campaign has been based on little scientific evidence and may have caused unintended health consequences."[106] Even worse, the horrible health consequences continue. Researchers know it and the data show it. In the next chapter, we'll look at the confusion at the heart of the low-fat and low-cholesterol myths.

It's All about Results: A Pragmatism Primer

Pragmatists are results-oriented—they believe something is right or wrong based on its results. People can try anything they want and the true worth of the program is revealed by its results. If it works, it is right. If it fails, it is wrong.

When it comes to weight loss, the pragmatic assessment would be based on the question: "Does the weight-loss program cause you to lose body fat and keep it off forever without compromising the rest of your life?" If so, then it is right. If not, then it is wrong. Unfortunately, this commonsense approach is not common practice. Despite the decades of data and tens of millions of overweight people that prove traditional weight-loss programs are wrong, those people have been brainwashed into thinking that they failed because they didn't lose any weight. But it's the weight-loss programs that have failed them. As Dr. Hilde Bruch of Baylor University puts it, "The efficacy of any treatment of obesity can be appraised only by the permanence of the result."[107] And by that metric, we don't have many programs that are doing so well.

Low-Fat, Low-Cholesterol
Confusion

Sugar-laden muffins, nutritionally neutered toast, and insulin-exploding juice are touted as part of a balanced, nutritious breakfast because they are low in fat. We look at any new food and ask ourselves, "Is this low in fat?" If the answer is yes, we think it is healthy. Yet foods that contain fat are not necessarily unhealthy.

Most researchers today agree that our total intake of fat is *not* a risk factor for cardiovascular disease or cancer. But don't low-fat diets help us lose weight? The Harvard School of Public Health strongly disagrees. "The low-fat, high-carbohydrate diet recommended by the ... USDA Food Guide Pyramid may be among the worst eating strategies for someone who is overweight. . . . People on low-fat diets generally lose about two to four pounds after several weeks, but then gain that weight back even while continuing with the diet. Randomized trials of weight loss usually show little net weight changes after a year." [108]

Foods containing fat do not make us fat, but we've been led to think so because a gram of fat contains more calories than a gram of carbohydrate or protein. Fat has 9 calories per gram while protein and carbohydrate have only 4. But as you've learned in earlier chapters, calories are not the primary issue—fat's higher quantity of calories does not mean eating fat causes us to store body fat. That thinking is rooted in the calorie-counting theory, which we know is wrong. International cholesterol expert Uffe Ravnskov, MD, PhD, puts it well: "The idea that you become fat by eating fat is just as silly as to say that you become green by eating green vegetables."[109]

According to the National Academy of Sciences, Harvard Medical School, Harvard School of Public Health, and dozens of other well-respected medical organizations, obesity itself is not associated with dietary fat in either national or international studies. No solid evidence proves that dietary fat or percentage of calories from fat causes weight gain. There is even evidence that *lower* fat intake correlates with *higher* obesity rates.

This evidence seems counterintuitive because we've been led to believe that eating whole-food fats encourages overeating. We've been misinformed.

Think back to Satiety. Water, fiber, and protein play the biggest role in the Satiety of food and Satiety determines how many calories we eat. Notice how there is no mention of fat there. Many water-, fiber-, and protein-packed foods contain fat. For example, seafood, meat, eggs, nuts, and seeds all contain a lot of fat. But when we focus on eating less fat, we replace these high-Satiety foods with low-Satiety but low-fat starches and sweets. Since low-Satiety foods require more calories to fill us up, this swap causes us to eat more—not fewer—calories. So,

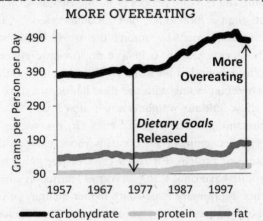

LESS NATURAL FOODS CONTAINING FAT, MORE OVEREATING

LESS NATURAL FOODS CONTAINING FAT, MORE BODY FAT

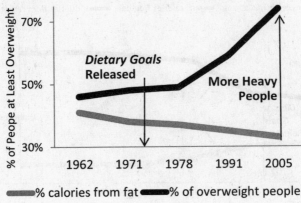

far from discouraging overeating, avoiding SANE foods that contain fat *encourages* overeating and hormonal clogging.

The last four decades of data tell the same story. We were told to avoid eating fat, so we reduced our relative intake of fat, increased our intake of starches and sweets, and were less satisfied. To deal with our

HOW WE EAT VERSUS OUR INCIDENCE OF WEIGHT GAIN

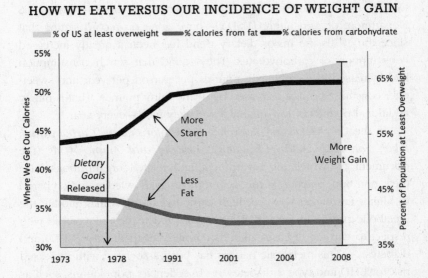

HOW WE EAT VERSUS OUR INCIDENCE OF DIABETES

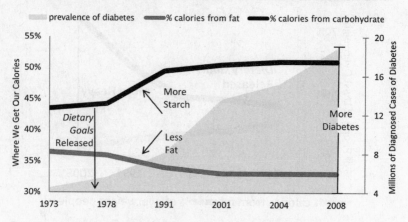

increased hunger we increased our total inSANE caloric intake and ended up sicker and heavier—albeit only a tiny fraction heavier relative to what we should have gained thanks to our set-point—as a result.

The government knows this too. The Centers for Disease Control and Prevention (CDC) reported, "During 1971–2000, a statistically significant increase in average energy intake occurred. . . . The increase in energy intake is attributable primarily to an increase in carbohydrate intake." [110] Even the authors of the government's guidelines—with the US Department of Agriculture (USDA)—have gone on record stating that since the 1970s the major dietary trend has been a greatly increased consumption of carbohydrates. They found that starch consumption had increased by nearly sixty pounds per person per year and sweetener consumption had increased by nearly thirty pounds. That is ninety additional pounds of low-quality low-Satiety food—every year.

In the USDA's *Dietary Reference Intakes for Energy, Carbohydrate, Fiber, Fat, Fatty Acids, Cholesterol, Protein, and Amino Acids* (the document on which all government and related organizations base their nutrition practices), the government acknowledges: "Compared to higher fat intakes, low fat, high carbohydrate diets may modify the metabolic profile in ways that are considered to be unfavorable with respect to chronic diseases such as coronary heart disease (CHD) and diabetes. . . . This metabolic pattern has been associated with increased risk for CHD and type 2 diabetes. . . . In sedentary populations, such as that of the United States where overweight and obesity are common, high carbohydrate, low fat diets induce changes in lipoprotein and glucose/insulin metabolism in ways that could raise risk for chronic diseases."[111]

So if low-fat/high-carb is linked to everything we're trying to avoid, why is it being recommended to us?

New York University researchers remind us of the sad fact that "dietary guidelines necessarily are political compromises between what science tells us about nutrition and health and what is good for the food industry."[112]

The emphasis on low fat leads away from eating SANE whole foods and misses an important point. Long-term health and fat loss do not result from diets low in fat, carbohydrate, or protein. Fat is not evil. Carbohydrates are not bad. And protein is not dangerous. The best way to burn body fat is to be balanced and SANE.

However, when you look at the government's pyramid and plate, balance is nowhere to be found:

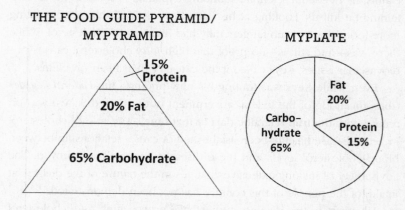

THE FOOD GUIDE PYRAMID/
MYPYRAMID

15%
Protein

20% Fat

65% Carbohydrate

MYPLATE

Fat
20%

Carbo-
hydrate
65%

Protein
15%

How are these balanced diets? They are high in carbohydrate and low in everything else. Consider the high-fat Atkins Diet. It is called "high-fat" because it advises individuals to get 65 percent of their calories from fat. Look at the USDA's pyramid and plate diets that advise us to get 65 percent of our calories from carbohydrate. Doesn't that make them high-carbohydrate diets? This could be why *USA Today* poked fun at the 72 percent of Americans who claimed to eat a balanced diet. The implication: "How could 70 percent of you be overweight if you ate a balanced diet?"[113] We could easily be overweight if the "balanced" diet we are told to eat by the government is actually out of balance.

This imbalance exists in other guidelines as well. The American Heart Association Nutrition Committee refers to a diet consisting of 40 percent carbohydrate, 30 percent fat, and 30 percent protein as a "low-carbohydrate/very-high-protein diet."[114] Since when does 40:30:30 indicate that anything is very high?

What could be the reason for this confusion? The answer lies in another myth that has been proved false: eating foods that contain fat leads to unhealthy cholesterol levels. The fact is that eating the right kinds of whole-food fats is key to improving our cholesterol.

WHOLE-FOOD FAT HELPS CHOLESTEROL

As with other popular misconceptions about how our bodies work, confusion runs rampant about the word "cholesterol." Ancel Keys played an important role in creating this problem. Along with his other claims, he needed a scientific-sounding explanation for how foods containing fat kill us. Looking at his data, Keys noticed that people eating more foods that contain fat generally had higher total cholesterol. While there was—and still is—no proof that high *total* cholesterol causes cardiovascular issues, Keys called it the cause of their heart problems.

Even while Keys was touting his new findings, the *Federal Register* (the official log of the federal government of the United States) was on record with the true scientific data at that time: "The role of cholesterol in heart disease has not been established. A causal relationship between blood cholesterol levels and these diseases has not been proved. The advisability of making extensive changes in the nature of the dietary fat intake of the people of this country has not been demonstrated."[115]

Likewise, to this day, no studies have proven high *total* cholesterol causes heart disease. The *American Journal of Medicine* reported, "Total cholesterol per se is not a risk factor for coronary heart disease at all."[116] Researcher Uffe Ravnskov, MD, PhD, analyzed twenty-six randomized and controlled trials, which were designed to lower total cholesterol and, theoretically, the risk of heart disease and of death from heart disease. Ravnskov's analysis divided people into two groups:

Treatment Group: People who ate less food that contains fat and/or took cholesterol-lowering drugs.

Control Group: People who did not eat less food that contains fat and did not take cholesterol-lowering drugs.

Across the studies, the total number of heart attack deaths was equal between the groups, and during the period of the trials *more* people died overall in the group who ate *less* fat and/or took cholesterol-lowering drugs.

Average Outcomes across the Twenty-Six Studies

	Treatment Groups	Control Groups
Fatal Heart Attacks	2.9%	2.9%
Total Death Rate	6.1%	5.8%

Ravnskov concluded: "Lowering serum cholesterol concentrations does not reduce mortality and is unlikely to prevent coronary heart disease."[117]

To prove that our government's dietary recommendations are helpful, three points must be proved:

1. Eating natural foods that contain fat leads to risky levels of cholesterol.
2. These levels of cholesterol cause heart disease.
3. The diet outlined by government's guidelines improves these cholesterol levels.

None of these things have been proved.

Eating whole foods containing fat has never been proved to lead to risky levels of cholesterol. The effect of natural dietary fat on cholesterol has never been proved to cause heart disease. Studies have actually shown the opposite. The high-starch, low-fat, and low-protein diet promoted by the government's guidelines has been proved to *worsen* the type of cholesterol (high-density lipoprotein, HDL) that decreases the risk of heart disease. For example, a 2009 study published in the *New England Journal of Medicine* went so far as to call HDL cholesterol "a biomarker for dietary carbohydrate."[118] In other words, the more "low-fat" carbohydrate we eat the lower our levels of the type of cholesterol that *is* crucial to heart health.

Here is where the confusion about cholesterol comes up: there are different types of cholesterol and most of them are helpful or neutral. The two most commonly discussed are LDL (low-density lipoprotein) and HDL. They are required to produce new cells and hormones. Because of this critical role, even if we never ate any cholesterol, our liver or intestines would produce it as our body works to keep us in balance. Much as unhealthy levels of body fat indicate a disorder in automatic energy balance and unhealthy levels of blood sugar indicate a disorder in automatic insulin balance, unhealthy levels of cholesterol indicate a disorder in automatic lipoprotein balance.

When it comes to predicting heart health, the American Heart Association, the International Diabetes Federation, and the World Health Organization agree that *low* HDL cholesterol—not *high* LDL cholesterol—is what matters. Looking at disease and death rates at various levels of LDL and HDL cholesterol, researchers have found that people with *low* HDL run a much greater risk of heart disease.

Relative Risk of Heart Disease[119]
(Total Cholesterol in Parenthesis)

	100 mg/dl LDL	160 mg/dl LDL	220 mg/dl LDL
85 mg/dl HDL	Very Low (185)	Very Low (245)	Very Low (305)
65 mg/dl HDL	Low (165)	Low (225)	Moderate (285)
45 mg/dl HDL	Low (145)	Moderate (205)	High (265)
25 mg/dl HDL	Moderate (125)	High (185)	Very High (245)

There are two things to note. First, *total* cholesterol is irrelevant. If people tell you their *total* cholesterol is 185, what is their risk of heart disease? Looking at the preceding table, it is either very low or high, depending on how much of that 185 consists of HDL cholesterol. Similarly, if people tell you their *total* cholesterol is 245, they either have a herculean heart or have a hemorrhaging heart, depending on their HDL levels.

Second, note how increasing HDL cholesterol is more important for heart health than decreasing LDL cholesterol. High HDL cholesterol protects us from heart problems more than dropping our LDL levels ever could. Heart-healthy diets are not about lowering *total* cholesterol. They are about raising HDL cholesterol.

The most effective way to raise our HDL levels through diet is to eat more whole-food fat and less starch. Whole-food fat raises HDL. Starch lowers HDL.

THE IMPACT OF FAT AND STARCH ON CHOLESTEROL AND HEALTH

	HDL	LDL	Health Impact
Unsaturated Fats (most plants, seafood, white meat)	↑	↓	☺☺
Saturated Fats (coconut, cocoa, dark/red meat)	↑	↑	☺
Starch (grains, corn, potatoes)	↓	↓	☹

Since lower HDL does more harm than lower LDL does good, any diet that tells us to replace SANE sources of fat with inSANE starch worsens our cholesterol. That's why many experts, from researchers at Harvard to scientists reporting in the *Journal of the American Medical Association*, believe our focus on eradicating fat (especially saturated fat) to try to reduce our LDL and total cholesterol may not just have failed to reduce heart disease risk—it may actually have increased it, along with decreasing our health, weakening our blood sugar control, and increasing the prevalence of insulin resistance and obesity.

Even saturated fats, about which so much has been said, are not cholesterol criminals. The American Heart Association found that no well-designed randomized controlled study in the general population has shown that lowering saturated fat intake significantly decreases our risk of coronary heart disease mortality.

Let's also keep in mind the critical benefits of whole-food fats. Our bodies can't make much use of vitamins A, D, E, K, and quite a few other helpful substances unless we eat fats. This is why your multivitamin instructs you to "take with a meal." The manufacturers are hoping your pill will find some natural fats to help the vitamins get where they need to go. Dietary fat also plays a critical role in cell and hormone production as well as brain function. Certain saturated fats known as medium-chain triglycerides (such as those in coconuts) and polyunsaturated fats known as omega-3 fatty acids (such as those in fish, flaxseed, chia seeds, and grass-fed beef) are especially helpful for heart and brain health and have been shown to help us burn body fat. We should see these whole-food fats as health foods rather than the cause of arterial clogs.

Please disregard the performances on commercials and talk shows that demonstrate that saturated fats are solid at room temperature and tell you that this is why they get clogged in our arteries. By that logic spinach, broccoli, and all other vegetables also get clogged in our arteries, as they are also solid at room temperature.

We know the cause of clogs. They do not come from whole-food fats. They come from starches and sweets. The *Journal of the American Medical Association* summarized the science beautifully: "The proportion of total energy from fat appears largely unrelated to risk of cardiovascular disease, cancer, diabetes, or obesity. Saturated fat—targeted by nearly all nutrition-related professional organizations and governmental agencies—has little relation to heart disease within most prevailing dietary patterns."[120]

What is the bottom line? The overwhelming evidence shows that any diet telling you to replace whole-food fats with starches is unhealthy and fattening.

Sadly, the government's diet tells us to do exactly what science says we should avoid.

If you think this is troubling, wait until you see what happened when big business jumped onto the government bandwagon.

Why Good Health Is Bad Business

We all know that Washington, DC, is home to many lobbyists. None of us like how much influence they have over our elected officials, yet we somehow overlook the fact that some of the largest lobbying efforts in the country are made by firms representing the food industry.

The days of family-run farms growing our crops are long gone. Today our food is grown by huge agribusiness concerns. According to a 2007 report by doctors Mary Hendrickson and William Heffernan, of the Department of Rural Sociology at the University of Missouri, 83.5 percent of beef, 80 percent of soybeans, and 55 percent of flour are produced by the top four firms in those industries. A single company supplies the seeds for 90 percent of genetically modified corn and soybeans.

Or consider the dairy industry. Not all dairy products are inSANE, but how did dairy products end up with their own food group while becoming a "required" part of a "balanced" diet? Might the $1.4 billion dollars spent on agribusiness lobbying have played a part?

That's why we need to watch where we get our nutrition information. Is the source driven by science or profits? When the answer is profits, we hear things like this from the Grocery Manufacturers of America—the people responsible for ensuring grocery stores are as profitable as possible: "Policies that declare foods 'good' or 'bad' are counterproductive." [121] A similar platitude is offered by the National Soft

Drink Association: "As refreshing sources of needed liquids and energy, soft drinks represent a positive addition to a well-balanced diet."[122]

None of these statements are backed by science. Again, we will not become clogged if we treat ourselves to starch and soda occasionally. But starch and sweets should never be *recommended* as part of a "balanced" diet. Food corporations know better than anyone else what the facts are, but they are not going to condemn themselves. Quite the opposite. Food companies aggressively fight any scientific information that threatens their bottom line.

Sadly, the crowding out of sound science by money doesn't stop there. Nearly two thirds, or 64 percent, of the members of national committees on nutrition and food receive compensation from food companies. David Willman at the *Los Angeles Times* reported that "at least 530 government scientists at the National Institutes of Health, the nation's preeminent agency for medical research, have taken fees, stock, or stock options from biomedical companies in the last five years."[123] Both the food industry and our government are paid to keep profits high, not to teach us about nutritional science. Don't forget the old adage, "It is hard to get people to believe one thing when they are paid to believe another."

SWEETENERS: MORE PROFITABLE, COMMON, AND DANGEROUS THAN EVER

The most common and powerful weapon in the food industry's arsenal is added sweeteners. The problem has gotten so bad that at the turn of the millennium the average American ate over 150 pounds of sweeteners per year because food companies add them to at least the following products:

baked or processed foods	protein bars
almost anything not refrigerated	low-fat salad dressing
low-calorie snacks	dairy products
"weight-loss" products	cough syrups
beverages	

Thanks to this sweet saturation, the average American is eating a little under a half pound of added sweeteners *per day*. That is a cup of clog every single day. Two centuries ago, people ate about one-tenth of that. During the previous 99.8 percent of our evolution, our ancestors ate none.

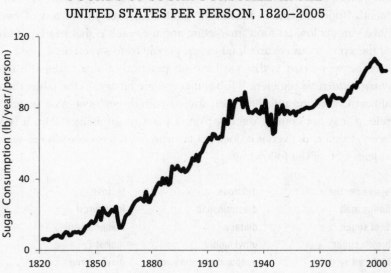

POUNDS OF SUGAR CONSUMED IN THE UNITED STATES PER PERSON, 1820–2005

Source: Stephan J. Guyenet, PhD, and Jeremy Landen, http://wholehealthsource.blogspot.com/2012/02/by-2606-us-diet-will-be-100-percent.html.

As early as the 1950s, Barry Popkin, PhD, of the University of North Carolina at Chapel Hill, pointed out that the research "link between sugar consumption and coronary heart disease . . . was stronger than

A Note about Sweeteners

When I talk about sweeteners, I am talking about sweeteners containing calories that are added to foods: substances like sugar, high-fructose corn syrup, evaporated cane juice, etc. I am not talking about the sugars already found in natural foods like fruits. Those are fine for many people. I am also not talking about natural calorie-free sweeteners like stevia. Those are fine. I'm also not talking about artificial calorie-free sweeteners such as aspartame, sucralose, or saccharin. Those are not good, but are preferable to sugar or high-fructose corn syrup.

the link between heart disease and the consumption of saturated fats from animal foods."[124] This work, however, was ignored.

How did this inSANEity happen? Food that has all its fat removed doesn't taste very good. It is hard to sell bad-tasting food. So food companies add sweeteners when they remove fat. Combine the government's "food containing fat is evil" guidelines with $36 billion of "we have yummy low-fat food" marketing and the result is that nearly a fifth of the average American's total calories come from sweeteners.

The worst part is that we have no practical choice under the *Dietary Guidelines* regimen. If foods that contain fat are off the table, then almost everything else has been stuffed with sweeteners. As a general rule, if it is not coming directly from a plant or an animal, then it has been sweetened. Even if it does not taste sweet, it has been altered with at least one of the following:

agave nectar	dextrose	lactose
barley malt	diastatic malt	malt syrup
beet sugar	diatase	maltodextrin
brown sugar	ethyl maltol	maltose
buttered syrup	evaporated cane juice	maple syrup
cane crystals	fructose	molasses
cane-juice crystals	fruit juice	muscovado sugar
cane sugar	fruit-juice concentrates	panocha
caramel	galactose	raw sugar
carob syrup	glucose	refiner's syrup
castor sugar	glucose solids	rice syrup
confectioner's sugar	golden sugar	sorbitol
corn sweetener	golden syrup	sorghum syrup
corn syrup	granulated sugar	sucrose
corn-syrup solids	grape sugar	sugar
crystalline fructose	high-fructose corn syrup	syrup
date sugar	honey	treacle
demerara sugar	icing sugar	turbinado sugar
dextran	invert sugar	yellow sugar

Memorizing this list isn't necessary—just know that *any* form of caloric sweetener causes clogs. Our body does not care where we get caloric sweeteners. To our body, apple juice is basically the same as soda, since they both contain about thirty grams of sugar per cup. A "weight-loss" bar with thirty grams of sweeteners in it causes the same clog as a candy bar of the same size with thirty grams of sugar in it. And watch out for misleading "natural" marketing. Unnatural high-fructose corn syrup (HFCS) has been rightfully demonized, owing in part to its high fructose content (42 percent). However, the supposedly "healthy" natural replacement agave nectar contains more than twice the amount of fructose (90 percent). Sure the juice, bar, cereal, and agave may have some additional accompanying nutrients, but that doesn't make the sweeteners in them any less harmful. Dissolving a vitamin pill in a can of soda doesn't make the soda healthy.

High-fructose corn syrup is especially common in low-calorie and low-fat products and is especially fattening. Combine this with the recommendation to avoid calories and foods containing fat, and we end up unintentionally eating 10,475 percent more HFCS than we did in 1970.

Eating all that HFCS is particularly harmful. Rats and people fed fructose consistently get fatter and sicker than rats and people fed the exact same amount of other sugars. HFCS sabotages our ability to feel satisfied by other foods as well. HFCS does not have low Satiety—it has *negative* Satiety. HFCS leaves us hungrier than if we did not eat it, altering our baseline levels of Satiety hormones and driving us to eat more and more over time. HFCS consumption also has a negative impact on insulin and leptin and contributes to an elevated set-point.

Sadly, it gets worse.

ADDICTED TO ADDED SWEETENERS

Experts at major research institutions have been quickly amassing evidence about the addictive nature of sugar. Studies at Princeton University show that lab rats that were repeatedly given a high-sugar diet and then had it taken away from them experienced behavioral and brain chemistry changes that mirror withdrawal from drugs such as morphine or nicotine. Other studies have found that sugar dependence is similar to dependence on amphetamines. The evidence is piling up: sweeteners are addictive.

Seem like a stretch? Consider this: *The Diagnostic and Statistical Manual of Mental Disorders*, edition IV (DSM-IV), defines us as chemically dependent on a substance if we experience at least three of the following symptoms in twelve months:

Increased tolerance—needing more for the same effect

Withdrawal—significant negative impact if we stop

Overuse—consuming more than is intended to be consumed

Loss of control—having our behavior meaningfully influenced by the substance

Exceptional effort to obtain—going beyond what is reasonable to get it

Overprioritization—allowing its use to interfere with more important activities

Ignoring negative consequences—continuing use regardless of disproportionately negative consequences

Using those guidelines—have any of us ever experienced any of these symptoms in conjunction with our sweetener habits?

Withdrawal: Ever tried to give up caloric sweeteners altogether? If so, how did that feel? If not, give it a whirl and you will experience how deeply this substance affects your brain.

Overuse: As the University of Washington's Stephan Guyenet, PhD, tells us, "in 1822, we ate the amount of added sugar in one 12 ounce can of soda every five days, while today we eat that much sugar every seven hours." [125]

Exceptional effort to obtain: Ever waited in line for way too long at your favorite ice cream place or gone out of your way to obtain a sweet treat?

Overprioritization: Ever been late to an appointment or meeting so that you could run to Starbucks and get your caramel mocha frappuccino?

Common sense and science seem to show sugar addiction quite clearly, but couldn't we say the same thing for any type of food? The research says no. Nicole Avena, PhD, a professor at the University of Florida's Center for Addiction Research and Education, tells us that studies show caloric sweeteners are unique in their ability to trigger "a series of behaviors similar to the effects of drugs of abuse." [126] She continues: "These are categorized as 'bingeing,' meaning unusually large bouts of intake, opiate-like 'withdrawal' indicated by signs of anxiety

and behavioral depression, and 'craving' measured during sugar absti-
nence as enhanced responding for sugar. There are also signs of both
locomotor and consummatory 'cross-sensitization' from sugar to drugs
of abuse (i.e., animals fed sugar are more likely to consume amphet-
amine, cocaine, alcohol)."

This unique and terrifying behavior is due to caloric sweeteners'
distinctive ability to activate a set of brain and hormonal responses previously thought to be limited to highly regulated drugs. As Carlo Colantuoni, PhD, an investigator in the Basic Sciences Division of the Lieber
Institute, tells us, "An opioid-mediated [morphinelike] dependence on
sugar has been demonstrated at both the behavioral and neurochemical
level." [127] University of Florida researchers add, "Based on the observed
behavioral and neurochemical similarities between the effects of intermittent sugar access and drugs of abuse, we suggest that sugar, as common
as it is, nonetheless meets the criteria for a substance of abuse and may
be 'addictive' for some individuals when consumed in a 'binge-like' manner." [128] Put plainly by Bartley Hoebel, PhD, professor of psychology in
the Program in Neuroscience at Princeton University, "In summary, sugar
has the addictive-like properties of both a psychostimulant and an opiate
[common opiates include morphine, opium, and heroin]." [129]

I don't mean to scare you, but for many, understanding and freeing
oneself from sweetener addiction is literally a matter of life and death.
When you switch to SANE eating, you will temporarily feel you are
going through withdrawal because you are. It takes the body a couple
of weeks to overcome the chemical dependence caused by the sea of
sweeteners we have been led to eat. But the switch is worth the effort.
After all, who wants to be an addict?

SWEETENERS: THE NEXT CIGARETTES?

In 1998 Coca-Cola offered schools $10,000 to advertise Coke discount
cards to their students. Deeply in need of the funds, Greenbrier High
School in Augusta, Georgia, invited Coke employees to lecture in classes
and added the analysis of Coca-Cola to its chemistry curriculum. The
school went on to make all 1,230 students dress in red or white shirts and
to spell-out "Coke" while they snapped photos to send to Coke execs.

Considering how harmful and addictive sweeteners are, why was
the Coke stunt considered harmless fun while it would be illegal to do

the same thing with other harmful and addictive substances? Can you imagine a group of schoolkids being asked to create a live depiction of the Marlboro Man?

Researchers have proved that sweeteners and tobacco are both harmful and addictive. They've proved that sweeteners are to diabetes what smoking is to lung cancer. Yet the promotion of the former is encouraged while the promotion of the latter is highly regulated. The rationale cannot be that tobacco is so much more harmful. Tobacco kills only 8 percent more people. Both industries are even run by the same companies:

A BRIEF HISTORY OF BIG TOBACCO AND THE "FOOD" INDUSTRY

1970	Philip Morris buys Miller Brewing
1978	Philip Morris buys 97 percent of Seven-Up
1985	R.J. Reynolds buys Nabisco Foods
1985	Philip Morris buys General Foods
1988	Philip Morris buys Kraft, Inc.
1990	Philip Morris acquires Jacobs Suchard
1993	Philip Morris buys Nabisco cereals
2000	Philip Morris buys Nabisco Holdings

Sweeteners and tobacco are even rationalized the same way by industry insiders. Here is how both describe the safety of their products:

Tobacco	InSANE Food Products
"I believe nicotine is not addictive."	"Soft drinks do not cause pediatric obesity, do not reduce nutrient intake, and do not cause dental cavities."
—Philip Morris Tobacco Company president[130]	—National Soft Drink Association[131]

They share the same marketing tactics:

Tobacco	InSANE Food Products
"The base of our business is the high school student."	"We always, always have kid-related programs."
—Lorillard Tobacco Company[132]	—Vice President, McDonald's[133]

And finally, on health:

Tobacco	InSANE Food Products
"We believe the products we make are not injurious to health." —Tobacco Industry Research Committee[134]	"Actually, our product is quite healthy. Fluid replenishment is a key to health. . . . Coca-Cola does a great service because it encourages people to take in more and more liquids." —Coke's CEO[135]
"We accept an interest in people's health as a basic responsibility, paramount to every other consideration in our business." —Tobacco Industry Research Committee[136]	"The soft drink industry has a long commitment to promoting a healthy lifestyle for individuals— especially children." —The National Soft Drink Association[137]

Since tobacco and sweeteners have so much in common, it seems odd that one of these is treated like the plague while it is fine for the food industry to spend hundreds of millions of dollars per year advertising sweets to children—particularly when psychologists have shown that before the age of eight, children do not see commercials as marketing; they see them as fact.

Consider the study from the *Journal of Marketing* that showed 70 percent of six- through eight-year-olds believe fast foods are healthier than food prepared at home. Kelly Brownell, PhD, former director of the Rudd Center for Food Policy and Obesity at Yale University, reports, "A study of Australian children ages nine to ten indicated that more than half believe that Ronald McDonald knows best what children should eat."[138] Brownell's research also reveals that the average American child sees ten thousand food advertisements each year, just on television. Children watching Saturday morning cartoons see a food commercial every five minutes. The vast majority are for sugared cereals, fast foods, soft drinks, sugary and salty snacks, and candy.

What's the moral of the story? Food companies are not going to stop with sweeteners. Nor can we rely on our government for help—it is the very source of the guidelines that leave us no practical choice other than to be slathered with sweeteners. Let's talk about how we can get our SANEity back.

Can SANE Eating and Smarter Exercise Save Your Life? Jim's Story

The story of seventy-year-old Jim is nothing short of remarkable. In Jim's words:

It started in 1959. I stood at my father's hospital bedside and watched while he suffered a fatal heart attack. It was also my sister's birthday. She was only 11 and my twin brother and I were 16. Dad was only 39 and I feared I would have the same fate. That memory still haunts me today. Don't worry, this story has a happy ending.

Fast-forward a few decades and I followed in my father's footsteps—suffering from a major heart attack at age 40. Then at age 63, my heart did its best to throw in the towel. However, my surgeon performed a quadruple bypass and my electrophysiologist installed an internal cardio defibrillator (ICD). The unit records all abnormal cardiac events and works to keep me alive if and when I go into fibrillation. That has happened two times since the device was installed.

A year later at age 64, I went into heart failure and started having daily events of tachycardia. I had low energy, sleep apnea, and chronic events of premature ventricular contractions (PVCs) that could not be controlled. Drugs helped somewhat but also caused hypotension and my energy was nil. My heart wanted to stop, I felt it, but I wasn't ready to stop.

Knowing something had to change and figuring I had little to lose, I discontinued all medications except baby aspirin, prayed my dad was watching over me, looked for answers elsewhere, and discovered SANE eating and smarter exercise. Within two days I was eating ten servings of green vegetables; eating healthy protein and fats; giving up grains, starch, and sugar; and starting eccentric and smarter interval training.

What happened next was nothing short of spectacular. I got stronger than I've been in decades while shedding 6 inches from my waist. My LDL cholesterol dropped from 220 to 165 and my blood pressure dropped from 150/90 to 110/70. The greatest improvement was a 90 percent reduction in PVCs (as counted on my ICD) and a 100 percent cure for sleep apnea. My energy is the highest it has been in 30 years. I feel fully alive for the first time in decades.

Now for the happy ending I promised. During a recent visit, my cardiologist downloaded data from my ICD and happily reported my events of ventricular tachycardia were *zero*. I happily suggested she start SANE eating and smarter exercise as a cure for heart disease; it certainly cured mine. She responded with a resounding "Will do!"

15

How Humanity Can
Achieve SANEity

How do we avoid all this inSANEity? We need to be pragmatic and ask: is there any way of eating that is proven to keep people free from obesity, diabetes, heart disease, and cardiovascular disease—the "diseases of civilization"?

Yes. We can eat the way we did before civilization. We can eat things we find directly in nature—vegetables, seafood, meat, eggs, fruits, nuts, and seeds—we can eat whole foods rich in water, fiber, and protein. It just makes sense. Why would anything or anyone "design" us to run on a low-fat/low-protein/high-starch diet that was not possible for 99.8 percent of our history? And if this sounds similar to paleo and primal diets, that's because it is. Paleo and primal diets high in nutrient-dense vegetables and low in starches and sweets are extremely SANE and effective. Remember, SANEity is used to enhance our existing lifestyle, not to do away with it.

The closer a food is to a plant we could gather or an animal we could hunt, the more SANE it is. And if anything other than cooking or cutting is required between the plant or animal and our stomach, then it probably does not belong in our stomach to begin with. This point has nothing to do with eating organic versus conventional food. Until someone discovers a Cheerios tree, a pasta plant, or a bread bush, conventional blueberries are more SANE than organic Cheerios, pasta, or bread. To quickly illustrate this idea, look at the chart below and circle how we obtain each of the foods listed. The answers are in the table footnote.

THE "IS IT ACTUALLY NATURAL?" QUIZ

Food	How Humans Get It		
Fruit	Process/Manufacture	Gather	Hunt
Bread	Process/Manufacture	Gather	Hunt
Rice	Process/Manufacture	Gather	Hunt
Vegetables	Process/Manufacture	Gather	Hunt
Seafood	Process/Manufacture	Gather	Hunt
Meat	Process/Manufacture	Gather	Hunt
Nuts	Process/Manufacture	Gather	Hunt
Seeds	Process/Manufacture	Gather	Hunt
Pasta	Process/Manufacture	Gather	Hunt
Sweets	Process/Manufacture	Gather	Hunt
Cereal	Process/Manufacture	Gather	Hunt
Eggs	Process/Manufacture	Gather	Hunt

Fruit: Gather. Bread: Process/Manufacture. Rice: Process/Manufacture. Vegetables: Gather. Seafood: Hunt. Meat: Hunt. Nuts: Gather. Seeds: Gather. Pasta: Process/Manufacture. Sweets: Process/Manufacture. Cereal: Process/Manufacture. Eggs: Gather.

Keep in mind that this is a general rule. There are exceptions. Some include low-sugar protein powders and bars, low-sugar jerkies, cottage cheese, and *plain Greek* yogurt. These foods are healthy sources of protein, so enjoy them even though they were not available to our ancestors. Electricity wasn't available to our ancestors either, but that doesn't mean we would be better off without it. On the other hand, even though starches such as potatoes, rice, and corn were available to our ancestors, these foods are best avoided, owing to their relatively low water, fiber, and protein content.*

Unless our metabolic system completely transformed itself in the last 0.02 percent of our evolutionary history—the twelve thousand years since we first started farming—filling our system with substances that it is not designed to digest will cause a clog. Dr. John Yudkin, of the

---

* One or two servings of sweet potatoes per week are fine.

University of London, notes that significant evolutionary adaptations of the human genome require between one thousand and ten thousand generations. "If there have been great changes in man's environment that occurred in a much shorter time," says Yudkin, "there are likely to be signs that man has not fully adapted, and this will probably show itself as the presence of disease."[139] More simply: We did not change, but the quality of our diet did. And this has left us heavy, diabetic, and sick.

A study from the University of Texas Southwestern Medical Center at Dallas showed that our modern diet increases nearly all the risk factors for the diseases of civilization when compared with a pre-starch-and-sweetener diet. Similar work at the Haimoto Clinic, Lund University, and Duke University Medical Center has shown a more natural diet to be the best diet available for clog clearing. In a University of Melbourne study, middle-aged Australian hunter-gatherers started out lean and free from type 2 diabetes, then switched to a diet inspired by the government's guidelines and became overweight and type 2 diabetic. Then they reverted back to their natural diet. In only seven weeks, the tribesmen lost an average of 16.5 pounds.

The list of studies proving the same results goes on, but Emory University researchers give us the bottom line: "Following a diet comparable to the one that humans were genetically adapted to should postpone, mitigate, and in many cases prevent altogether, a host of diseases that debilitate us."[140]

Let's turn next to how we can do that in detail.

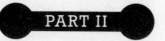

PART II

THE SOLUTIONS

To any woman out there who is fed up with trying the same thing over and over, I offer this suggestion. Instead of getting back on the treadmill "one more time," try this. Alter your diet so that you eat no grain-based carbohydrate: no flour, no sugar, no bread, no pasta, and no high-fructose corn syrup. Then go to the gym and perform a workout of leg press, pull down, chest press, row and overhead press. Lift slowly and smoothly but with as much effort as possible. Go to complete fatigue, or as close to it as you can tolerate. Work out once, or at most, twice a week. Make sure your workouts last no longer than 20 minutes. Then sit back and watch what happens.

—Doug McGuff, MD [141]

Go SANE with Your Diet

For the vast majority of people, being overweight is not caused by how much they eat but by what they eat. The idea that people get heavy because they consume a high volume of food is a myth. Eating large amounts of the right food is your key to success.

—Joel Fuhrman, MD, *Eat to Live*

A common assumption is that switching over to a healthier lifestyle means spending a lot more money and time on food. That's not true, at least not when you enjoy a SANE lifestyle. We'll focus on approaches that give us the most results with the least investment of time and money possible. We are going to focus on simplicity and practicality instead of perfection.

We can keep things simple by breaking down SANE eating into three components:

1. Nonstarchy Vegetables = SANE Carbohydrates
2. Nutrient-Dense Proteins = SANE Proteins
3. Whole-Food Fats/Low-Fructose Fruits = SANE Fats and Sweets

Please also keep in mind that SANE eating (and the Smarter exercise we will cover shortly) should be seen as a starting point, not an ending point. We all have unique situations and metabolisms and what works for some of us may not work for others. The key is having the information necessary to create a sustainable lifestyle that keeps

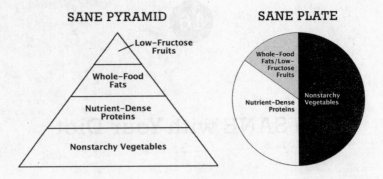

us happy and healthy. There is one right diet just as there is one right outfit—that is, there isn't one.

Finally, remember that the guidelines we will cover here are designed to help people like you develop excellent health along with a world-class physique. If your goals are more modest, then you don't need to follow these guidelines precisely. Do what works for you. The key is letting the scientific facts guide you. In my experience, for the majority of us, effort is not the issue. We've tried incredibly hard, but we've been given the wrong set of tools. Let's work on giving you the right toolbox to meet your goals.

The SANEity of Food Groups

Food Group	SANEity Rating	How Much to Eat
Nonstarchy Vegetables	★ ★ ★ ★	As much as you possibly can. 10+ servings per day, many of which are green, with (hopefully) some raw.
Nutrient-Dense Protein	★ ★ ★ ★ ★	More than most people currently do. 3–6 30- to 55-gram servings per day, totaling between 100 and 200 grams.
Whole-Food Fats	★ ★ ★ ⅃	More than most people currently do. 3–6 servings per day, especially seafood, cocoa/cacao, coconut, avocado, chia, and flax.
Low-Sugar Fruits	★ ★ ★ ⅃	More than most people currently do. 0–3 servings per day from berries/citrus.

Legumes	★ ★ ★	As needed. 0–2 servings per day.
High-Sugar Dairy	★ ★ ✓	As little as possible.
High-Sugar Fruits	★ ★ ✓	As little as possible.
Other Fats	★ ★	As little as possible.
Whole-Grain Starch	★ ✓	As little as possible.
Processed Starch	✓	None.
Sweeteners		None.

★ ★ ★ ★ ★	Excellent
★ ★ ★ ★	Great
★ ★ ★	Average
★ ★	Poor
★	Terrible
	Poison

Nutrients Provided by SANE Eating versus the Typical US Diet

	SANE	Typical US
Carbohydrate	Less	More
Sugar and Starch	Much less	Much more
Fruits	More	Less
Nonstarchy Vegetables	Much more	Much less
Protein	More	Less
Fat	Equal	Equal
Unnatural Trans Fats*	Much less	More
Natural Unsaturated Fat	More	Less
Natural Saturated Fat	Equal	Equal
Antioxidants	Much more	Much less
Fiber	Much more	Much less
Vitamins and Minerals	Much more	Much less
Body Fat Stored	Much less	More
Food Eaten	More	Less

*Unnatural fats engineered by food product manufacturers to decrease costs and increase shelf life. They are the high-fructose corn syrup of fats, and should be avoided.

Review the SANE row of the table above. I am not saying eat *more* for shock value. Researchers estimate that prior to the advent of starch and sweeteners, our ancestors ate up to five pounds of food per day. Thanks to all the water, fiber, and protein, SANE foods are literally larger in size than starches and sweets. Our shopping carts, refrigerators, and plates will be much fuller when we go SANE.

No more tiny, sweet, starchy breakfasts. You can have luscious omelets overflowing with nonstarchy vegetables and nutrient-dense protein, generous protein-packed smoothies, and SANE cereals (see recipes in chapter 25). No more flaccid sandwiches for lunch and soggy starch for dinner. Enjoy a double serving of delightful seafood or succulent nutrient-dense meat accompanied by a triple serving of nonstarchy vegetables. Finish up with a large chocolaty, nutty, creamy, or crunchy serving of a whole-food fat-rich SANE dessert and you will be satisfied and slim.

SANE Carbohydrates

Step one of going SANE: cover at least half of your plate with non-starchy vegetables. As a general rule, nonstarchy vegetables are the vegetables that you could eat raw. For example, corn, potatoes, and many root vegetables cannot be eaten raw. They are starches. Spinach, kale, romaine lettuce, broccoli, mushrooms, carrots, onions, and generally things you find in salads can be eaten raw and are nonstarchy vegetables. Even more generally, if it's a plant and you can't eat it raw (starchy vegetables, grains, and legumes), you are likely to be healthier and slimmer swapping it for a plant you could eat raw (nonstarchy vegetables, fruits, nuts, and seeds).

Both fresh and frozen nonstarchy vegetables are excellent choices. Sometimes frozen nonstarchy vegetables can be even better options as their fresh counterparts may not be fresh. Frozen vegetables are often flash frozen in their prime. This is useful because regardless of when you eat them you will enjoy a nearly optimal amount of nutrients. Fresh vegetables in their prime are wonderful options; just make sure they are actually in their prime. (Don't let them rot in the fridge!) Bottom line: Fresh and frozen nonstarchy vegetables should make up the majority of the food we eat.

Deep green vegetables such as spinach, kale, romaine lettuce, greens, broccoli, and so on are the best of the best when it comes to nonstarchy vegetables. Try to get the bulk of your nonstarchy vegetable intake from deep greens. The "deeply colored" rule also applies across the rainbow. With a few exceptions (such as cauliflower), the richer the color of the nonstarchy vegetable, the better it is for us. For example, light green iceberg lettuce isn't as healthy as the deeper green romaine lettuce, which lags behind very deep greens such as spinach or kale.

What about cooking? Our top priority is eating at least ten servings of nonstarchy vegetables per day, so do whatever is necessary within reason to get ten plus servings of nonstarchy vegetables into your body. (You'll find more tips on how to do that easily on page 211.) In an ideal world, most of your nonstarchy vegetables would be eaten raw to maximize nutrient and water content. But if you don't like them raw, that's fine. Again, raw is good, but eating more of them is even better.

With the exception of leafy green vegetables (spinach, kale, romaine lettuce, etc.) a serving is about the size of your fist or what fits in an eight-ounce measuring cup. A serving of raw leafy greens is two or three cups. If cooking makes the vegetables shrink (spinach, mushrooms, etc.), then a serving of the cooked nonstarchy vegetables is about half the size of your fist or half a cup.

Here are some examples of a single serving of nonstarchy vegetables:

6 asparagus spears	5 cherry tomatoes
8 baby carrots	5 sticks of celery
5 large broccoli florets	3 cups of raw leafy green vegetables
1 Roma tomato	½ cup of cooked spinach
4 slices of an onion	

Grocery List: Common Nonstarchy Vegetables (10+ Servings per Day)
Note: This is not an exhaustive list.

alfalfa sprouts	bok choy	chard	garlic
artichoke	broccoflower	chives	greens
arugula	broccoli	collards	green beans
asparagus	brussels sprouts	cucumber	kale
avocado	cabbage	dandelion greens	leaf amaranth
bean sprouts	carrots	eggplant	leeks
beets	cauliflower	endive	lemongrass
bell peppers	celery	escarole	mixed greens

mushrooms	peppers	shallot	sugar snap peas
mustard greens	pumpkin	snow peas	tomatoes
onion	romaine lettuce	spinach	turnip greens
parsley	sauerkraut	squash	zucchini

A SANE APPROACH TO CARBOHYDRATE

As you start going SANE, some uninformed individuals might accuse you of being on a low-carbohydrate diet—as if there's something wrong with being on a low-carb diet to begin with. There isn't. And you aren't.

The American Diabetes Association, the North American Association for the Study of Obesity, and the American Society for Clinical Nutrition made the following joint statement in their 2004 study in the journal *Diabetes Care*: "Glycemic [blood sugar/insulin] control was *better* with low-carbohydrate than with low-fat diet therapy in subjects with type 2 diabetes."[142] Similarly, an impressive two-year study published in the *New England Journal of Medicine* found that Mediterranean and low-carbohydrate diets are effective alternatives to the low-fat diet for weight loss and appear to be just as safe as the low-fat diet.[143] Not only is the SANEr approach to carbohydrates safe, but the experts found it more metabolically beneficial than the typical low-fat approach. Let's cover a few key points when thinking about "low-carb."

The single most important part of living a SANE lifestyle is eating *no less than ten servings of nonstarchy vegetables per day*. These types of vegetables are carbohydrates. Now, it might seem odd to call a lifestyle whose number one priority is eating as much of a certain type of carbohydrate as possible a low-carb diet. And it is similarly odd for people to claim that avoiding an extremely high-carb diet is a low-carb diet. What happened to medium-carb?

Low-carb dieters usually keep their carb count in the ballpark of 50 grams per day. A typical Western diet contains around 300 grams of carbohydrate per day. That's an extremely high-carb diet. The only way to fit 300 grams of carbohydrate into the human body is to consume concentrated and unSatisfying sources of carbohydrate, such as starches and sweets. When you go SANE, you will be too full for these forms of carbohydrate and will unconsciously consume between 70 and 125 grams of carbohydrate per day. You will avoid a diabetes- and obesity-inducing, extremely high-carb diet, but your carbohydrate count will not qualify you as a low-carb dieter.*

Much of this carbohydrate confusion comes from the fact that 90 percent of what we find in the grocery store is a carbohydrate. Defining carbohydrates as foods with most of their calories coming from carbohydrate, fats as foods with most of their calories coming from fat, and protein as foods with most of their calories coming from protein, we end up with:

Proteins	Fats	Carbohydrate
Seafood	Eggs	Everything else
Some meats	Tofu	
Egg whites	Oils	
Low-fat and low-sugar dairy	Nuts and seeds	
Low-sugar protein powders	Some meat	
	Full-fat dairy	

For example, the calories in whole milk come from 30 percent carbohydrate, 21 percent protein, and 49 percent fat. Whole milk is mostly fat, so it is a fat. The calories in skim milk come from 53 percent carbohydrate, 42 percent protein, and 5 percent fat. Skim milk is mostly carbohydrate, so it is a carbohydrate. How about the so-called "good source of protein," beans? They are 76 percent carbohydrate, 21 percent protein, and 3 percent fat. Beans are a carbohydrate. Broccoli is a carbohydrate with 71 percent of its calories coming from carbohydrate. So are bananas—93 percent carbohydrate. Grains, potatoes, rice, breads, pasta, beans, fruits, vegetables, and most dairy products are carbohydrates. Almost anything that doesn't need to be refrigerated or frozen (aside from oils, seasonings, etc., and nuts and seeds) and all sweet drinks are carbohydrates. However, many people think of carbohydrates as limited to starches and sweets. Given this incorrect view of nutrition, we can see why these people may mistakenly call us low-carb dieters.

---

* Note: This is not to imply that well-formulated low-carb/high-fat diets are unhealthy. Quite the opposite is true as we will see later. It is possible and healthy to go low-carb SANE, but "out-of-the-box" SANE eating does not qualify as low-carb.

The truth is that you and I will eat the SANEst carbohydrates in mass just as we eat the SANEst proteins and fats in mass. That doesn't make us low-carb dieters. That makes us healthy and slim.

THE LOW-CONFUSION/HIGH-NUTRITION DIET

I'm not fond of high- and low- labels. They generally do more harm than good. They polarize people who could be working together to help others avoid sweeteners, refined starches, and processed fats. But if we must slap a low- or high- diet label on our way of eating let's call it the low-confusion/high-nutrition diet.

I arrived at that title after considering four scientific facts:

1. **Vitamins and Minerals Are Essential.** We must eat vitamins and minerals or we get sick. For example, if you don't eat enough vitamin B_{12} (found only in animal products), you can develop a condition called hypocobalaminemia, which deteriorates the spinal cord and brain.

2. **Protein Is Essential.** We've all heard of essential amino acids. Amino acids are what our body turns protein into during digestion. Some amino acids are "essential" because if we do not eat them, we get sick.

3. **Fat Is Essential.** We've all heard of essential fatty acids. Fatty acids are what our body turns fat into during digestion. Some fatty acids are "essential" because if we do not eat them, we get sick.

4. **Carbohydrate Is NOT Essential.** None of us have heard of an essential carbohydrate. That's because there is no such thing. During digestion carbohydrate is converted into glucose. If we never ate any carbohydrate, we would not necessarily get sick, because our body would create glucose from other things we eat, such as protein.

I know that last fact may seem a bit controversial, but it's not. Even the carbohydrate-loving USDA noted it in its *Dietary Reference Intakes for Energy, Carbohydrate, Fiber, Fat, Fatty Acids, Cholesterol, Protein, and Amino Acids*:* "The lower limit of dietary carbohydrate compatible with life apparently is zero, provided that adequate amounts of protein and fat are consumed."[144] I am not sure why they stuck the word "ap-

---

* The document on which all things nutritional in the government and related organizations is based.

parently" in there, but oh well. The point is that there is no biological reason for a nonpower athlete (football player, sprinter, etc.) to eat carbohydrate unless it helps us to consume *required* vitamins, minerals, fat, or protein.

So why not forget about the high-carb, high-fat, and high-protein confusion and enjoy the foods that give us the most of what we need and the least of what we don't, and that kept us free from what ails us all long before anyone even uttered the word *calorie*? Long-term fat loss and health are not about high-carb, high-fat, or high-protein diets—they're about high-nutrition and low-confusion eating.

HOW SANEity COMPARES WITH COMMON DIETS

	Nonstarchy Vegetables	Low-Fructose Fruits	Nutrient-Dense Proteins	Whole-Food Fats	Most Dairy & Beans*	Oils	Starch	Added Sweeteners
Low-Carb	Medium	Low	High	Very High	Low	High	None	None
Typical US	Low	Low	Medium	Low	Medium	High	High	High
SANE	Very Very High	Medium to Low	High	Medium to High	Low	Low	None	None
Pyramid/ MyPlate	Medium	Medium	Low	Low	Medium	Low	Very High	Low
Low-Fat	Medium	Medium	Low	Low	Medium	None	Very High	Low

*Except for cheese. Low-carbohydrate diets generally encourage relatively high intakes of cheese.

Also, we can forget about simple carbohydrates versus complex carbohydrates. This distinction causes confusion. For example, SANE fruits contain simple carbohydrates, while inSANE starches contain complex carbohydrates. Oh no! Not so fast. The "healthy" complex carbohydrates rice, cereal, crackers, potatoes, and wheat bread are all *more* hormonally harmful (they all raise our blood sugar more) than the simple carbohydrate sugar. Let's avoid this complexity and enjoy more water-, fiber-, and protein-rich SANE plants and animals. The only form of carbohydrates in this category are nonstarchy vegetables and low-fructose fruits.

NONSTARCHY VEGETABLES: SANE CARBOHYDRATE SUMMARY

- Cover half of your plate with nonstarchy vegetables.
- If it can't be eaten raw, don't eat it.
- Stick with fresh or frozen.
- Greens are great.
- The deeper the color the higher the SANEity.
- Raw is ideal but not required.
- A serving is about one to three handfuls depending on how "dense" the nonstarchy vegetables are.
- Low-carb diets are great, but your SANE lifestyle doesn't have to be one.
- Ninety percent of what you see in a grocery store is carbohydrate.
- Carbohydrate is nonessential, so focus on carbs that carry along with them the most essential nutrients possible.

SANE Proteins

The second step to going SANE is filling a third of our plate with nutrient-dense protein. This ratio should ensure we get 30 to 55 grams of protein at each meal. In general, a serving size will be about as large as two of your palms. For example, a large piece of lean meat or fish, a cup and a half of cottage cheese or plain Greek yogurt, three eggs and a large piece of ham, eight egg whites, or a can of tuna.

It's important to aim for a minimum serving of about 30 grams of protein. If we consume less than this in a sitting we will not enjoy all the benefits protein has to offer. That's because when we eat 30 grams or more of protein, the concentration of a specific amino acid in our blood, called leucine, becomes high enough to cause our body to re-fresh and renew our lean tissue. The technical term for this is *muscle protein synthesis*—our body is rebuilding itself, and without activat-ing this mechanism at least three times a day, we are missing out on all sorts of metabolic benefits and risk losing about 5 percent of our muscle tissue per decade. This condition is known as sarcopenia, can be thought of as osteoporosis for muscles, and is easily avoided if we take a SANE approach to protein.

We will be consuming more nutrient-dense protein than the com-mon RDA, or recommended daily allowance. This is because the com-mon RDA is what we need to eat if our goal is to avoid malnutrition. Our goal isn't to avoid malnutrition. Our goal is to enjoy robust health and leanness throughout our life.

To do this, eat 30- to 55-gram servings of protein at least three times per day. Aim for a total of between 100 grams and 200 grams of protein per day depending on your size and activity level. A five-foot-tall 110-pound sedentary woman would be fine with about 100 grams, while a six-foot-tall 195-pound man who exercises smarter should take in about 200 grams. If you follow the serving guides, tips, and recipes we'll cover, and enjoy nutrient-dense protein every time you eat, you will achieve this easily and be surprised at how full you are and how much better you feel and look long term. Researchers at Maastricht University in the Netherlands have found that additional protein consumption results in a significantly lower body weight regain after weight loss.*

When we talk about eating protein, many people immediately think of meat. Nutrient-dense meat is a great source of protein; however, seafood is also a wonderful source of protein. A flood of research suggests that in addition to all the protein-related benefits already discussed, consuming seafood frequently can drop our risk of the vast majority of diseases plaguing us today. Do your best to eat seafood daily. Not a few times per week. Daily. This is simple because cooking seafood is a snap. Place some fish and some seasoning in a pan or baking dish and heat it. You will be delighted when you eat it. Canned seafood options such as canned salmon, tuna, and sardines require no cooking and provide inexpensive portable protein.

When considering protein options, keep in mind that just because a food has some protein in it, this does not qualify it as a useful source of protein. Not all proteins are created equal, and many of the "good sources of protein" we hear of are about as good at meeting our protein needs as ketchup is good at meeting our nonstarchy vegetable needs.

Let's define concentrated sources of protein as common foods that have more calories coming from protein than from fat or carbohydrates, and whose protein can be readily used by the body.

---

* Note: When thinking about grams of protein keep in mind that—for example—a 200-gram serving of salmon contains about 40 grams of protein. Like most SANE foods, salmon is mostly water. We are aiming for between 100 and 200 grams of *protein*, not 100 to 200 grams of foods containing protein; we'll be enjoying far more delicious food than that.

Concentrated Sources of Protein
seafood: 51% to 94% protein
egg whites: 91% (this isn't about fearing fat; details coming)
white meat with or without skin: 51% to 80% protein
dark meat without skin: ~60% protein
low-fat cottage cheese: 60% to 85% protein (same fat disclaimer as above)
low-fat plain Greek yogurt: 60% to 70% protein (ditto)
lean (ideally grass-fed) red meat: 51% to 75% protein (ditto)
low-sugar casein or whey protein powder: >70% protein

There are also a few fairly concentrated sources of protein. They are given that designation because quite a few of their calories come from fat or carbohydrate and, for the plant options, they do not contain an optimal set of amino acids and are not as readily used by the body. None of these things are deal breakers. Especially if the calories are coming from natural fats. Natural fats are great for us. But let's be honest. If 63 percent of the calories in an egg comes from fat while only 35 percent comes from protein, eggs are not a concentrated source of protein. Again, that is fine. Eggs are SANE. But it does not make sense to call something that is mostly fat or carbohydrate a concentrated source of protein. Pretty good is reasonable, though.

Fairly Concentrated Sources of Protein
dark-meat poultry with skin: ~45% protein
moderately fatty (ideally grass-fed) red meat: 40% to 60% protein
eggs: 35% protein
soybeans: 33% protein
low-sugar vegetarian protein powders (rice, pea, hemp): >50% protein

Everything else is not even close to being a concentrated source of protein. Common dairy products other than those listed are mostly fat and sugar. Beans are mostly carbohydrate. Nuts are more than 70 percent fat. Again, being mostly fat or carbohydrate does not necessarily make these foods bad; it just makes it inaccurate to call them concentrated sources of protein.

Now, about those "low-fat" disclaimers in the list of concentrated sources of protein. Given all the science showing that we should not fear whole-food fats, some people get justifiably concerned when they hear anything about *low-fat* cottage cheese, *low-fat* plain Greek yogurt, *lean* cuts of meat, and egg *whites*. Let's clarify. When we're talking about *nutrient-dense* proteins, we're talking about foods with as much protein, vitamins, and minerals *per calorie* as possible. If you have two instances of a food that are the same in every way except that one contains more fat than the other (for example, fat-free versus full-fat cottage cheese), divide the protein, vitamins, and minerals in a serving by the calories in a serving and the option with less fat is the more nutrient-dense source of protein. This is not to say that the full-fat versions of these foods should be avoided. It's to say that if your goal is to pick a food that maximizes protein, vitamin, and mineral intake, this is done by picking leaner options. Natural fats are wonderful for us. But we're talking about how to eat protein, not how to eat fat. We'll cover fat in a moment.

Speaking of nutrition-minded communities, some vegetarians and vegans may have something to say to you about protein. We'll cover the science pertaining to meat shortly, but please keep in mind that vegetarians and vegans can enjoy a Satisfying, unAggressive, Nutritious, and inEfficient lifestyle as much as anyone else. Replacing starches and sweets with nonstarchy vegetables, nutrient-dense protein, whole-food fats, and low-fructose fruits is as healthy and slimming for those who eat animal products as it is for those who abstain.

The wrinkle for vegetarians and vegans has to do with a point mentioned earlier: "Not all proteins are equal." One of the major reasons we need to eat protein is that we need to eat certain amino acids. Not all proteins are the same when it comes to the quality and quantity of essential amino acids they provide. Animal products provide much better essential amino acid "profiles" than plant products. Animal sources of protein are also more easily utilized by the body. Again, it is possible to consume a SANE quantity and quality of protein without eating animal products. However, it is much easier if we enjoy seafood, organ meats, grass-fed red meat, poultry, lean conventional red meat, eggs, cottage cheese, and plain Greek yogurt. If these high-quality and healthy options are off the table, protein powders made from rice, pea, or hemp protein are good substitutions. I also advise vegetarians to take a branched-chain amino acid supplement to address the suboptimal amino acid profile of plants.

A SANE APPROACH TO PROTEIN

Eating at least three 30- to 55-gram servings of high-quality and nutrient-dense protein per day is the second most important aspect of our lifestyle. High-Satiety protein fills us up, keeps us full, and enables our body to preserve muscle tissue and burn fat instead of burning both. Finally, trading processed fats, starches, and sweets for nutrient-dense protein has been shown in a mountain of studies to improve nearly every aspect of our health. Donald Layman, PhD, professor of nutrition at the University of Illinois, determined that protein-rich diets can preserve muscle loss at less than 15 percent (or even zero, when the diet is combined with exercise) during weight loss. Increasing the proportion of protein to carbs especially helps women improve their body composition, their cholesterol and triglyceride levels, their blood sugar balance, and their Satiety as they lose weight. Finally, in the *American Journal of Clinical Nutrition*, Layman laid it all out:

> High-protein, low-carbohydrate diets have been found to have positive effects on reducing risk factors for heart disease, including reducing serum triacylglycerol, increasing HDL cholesterol, increasing LDL particle size, and reducing blood pressure. . . . High-protein, low-carbohydrate diets have also been investigated for treatment of type 2 diabetes with positive effects on [blood sugar control], including reducing fasting blood glucose, [post-meal] glucose and insulin responses, and the percentage of glycated hemoglobin [HbA1c, or, as we know it here, the hormonal clog].[145]

But alas, the better something is, the more vocal the misinformed extremists who embody the immortal saying, "Weak point, yell loud." And there is certainly some weak logic and loud yelling by those who embrace the traditional food pyramid view of protein consumption.

For instance, some misinformed individuals claim that eating a SANE amount of protein hurts the kidneys and liver. This assertion is not borne out in randomized controlled testing, say experts from Harvard to Finland. On the other hand, hundreds of studies show positive health benefits and body-fat loss stemming from the protein intake we're discussing. A typical report from Colorado State University (at www.catalystathletics

.com/articles/downloads/proteinDebate.pdf) cites the large body of experimental evidence that demonstrates a higher intake of lean animal protein reduces the risk for cardiovascular disease, hypertension, dyslipidemia, obesity, insulin resistance, and osteoporosis while not impairing kidney function. Researchers have shown that humans evolved to get about a third of our calories from protein—which means the so-called very-high-protein diets (30 percent to 40 percent total energy) are closer to the conditions that spawned our present-day human genome. How could a basic part of human evolution harm rather than help us? Emory University researchers made the point well when they noted, "It would be paradoxical if humans . . . should now somehow be harmed as a result of protein intake habitually tolerated or even required by their near relatives."[146] Rather than be helped, our health might actually be negatively affected if our dietary intake of protein fell *outside* this range.

In speaking about one of the most informative prospective health studies of all time, the Nurses' Health Study, Walter Willett, chair of the Harvard School of Public Health, shared a finding that the group of women who ate the most protein were 25 percent less likely to have had a heart attack or to have died of heart disease—so clearly, "eating a lot of protein doesn't harm the heart."[147]

With such clear scientific data, why do some books and documentaries continue to paint a bleaker picture of protein? Many of these resources confuse proven health benefits with moral or environmental concerns. They also often misrepresent data from the large observational study the China-Cornell-Oxford Project—popularized by the book *The China Study*.[148] For example, the data in this study show the consumption of nutrient-dense fish and meat, as well as eggs, correlating with a *lower* incidence of heart disease, while starchy plants that cannot be eaten raw correlate with a *higher* incidence of heart disease. In fact, a Harvard Medical School researcher went so far as to note that "wheat was by far the most toxic food found in the China Study."[149] Willett concludes, "A survey of 65 counties in rural China, however, did not find a clear association between animal product consumption and risk of heart disease or major cancers."[150] Even T. Colin Campbell, the author of *The China Study*, when reporting on his observations concerning fish consumption in China, noted that "it is the largely vegetarian, inland communities who have the greatest all risk mortalities and morbidities."[151]

The point here is not to criticize SANE plant-based diets. In fact, a SANE lifestyle *is* plant-based. Our plates will be filled with mostly non-starchy vegetables and a large chunk of our calories will come from plant fats such as cocoa, coconut, avocado, flax, and chia. The point is that we're talking about proven biology, not correlations, politics, or morality. Randomized controlled trials—the studies that provide the most definitive proof possible—show that health and fitness are maximized by eating water-, fiber-, and protein-rich foods.* These foods come from *both* plants and animals. As Joel Fuhrman, MD, states elegantly in his article "What You Need to Know about Vegetarian or Vegan Diets," "You can achieve the benefits of a vegetarian diet, without being a vegetarian or a vegan."[152]

So how did the myth that protein is bad for us get started in the first place? Apparently, the myth arose from studies in which animals were fed extreme amounts of low-quality sources of protein and then experienced problems. But rather than proving protein is harmful, these studies led to the discovery that until an inactive person exceeds 2 grams of protein per pound of body weight per day, we will get only healthier and slimmer by enjoying additional nutrient-dense proteins.

To put 2 grams of protein per pound of body weight into perspective, an inactive 150-pound person would not enter the protein-risk zone until he ate eleven chicken breasts per day, every day. That would total 2 grams of protein per pound of body weight and would mean that about 60 percent of his total calories were coming from protein. I think we can all agree that's not a good idea. Bad things happen if we eat too much of anything.

Luckily, it is impossible to consistently eat too much whole-food, nutrient-dense protein. Our stomach would explode before we did it. Worrying about eating too much whole-food nutrient-dense protein is a bit like worrying about drinking too much water. Can it be done? Yes. Will we do it? No.

---

* Observational studies such as the China-Cornell-Oxford Project provide us only with correlation, not causation. For instance, increased usage of sunglasses correlates with sunny days. That does not prove that wearing sunglasses causes the sun to come out.

Well, what about meat—if one listens to the mainstream media, it's hard not to come to the conclusion that something about meat must be unhealthy. While some might argue against eating meat for environmental or ethical reasons, science proves there is nothing inherently unhealthy about *nutrient-dense* meat. In fact, low levels of animal protein have been associated with an *increased* risk of strokes. Nutrient-dense meat was a cornerstone of our diet for most of our evolutionary history and there are no randomized controlled data showing that it is unhealthy. Academic work that cautions against meat is referring to the inSANE heavily processed meat such as hot dogs, baloney, pink slime, and so on, or to diets in which people replace vitamin- and mineral-rich foods with non-nutrient-dense meat. These works are quite right—we should not do either of those things. We should eat the most nutrient-dense food possible—and that includes many forms of seafood and meat. If you have any doubts, consider the *Journal of the American Medical Association*'s review of 147 diet and health studies.[153] That review found zero correlation between meat consumption and heart disease.

Nutrient-dense meat is not unhealthy. In fact, it is a fantastic source of essential protein, fat, vitamins, and minerals, and it promotes hormonal health. According to researcher James O'Keefe, MD, at the Mid America Heart and Vascular Institute, eating a good amount of lean protein at regular intervals can help you feel satisfied, increase your metabolic rate, improve your cholesterol ratio and your insulin sensitivity, and help speed weight loss as it also ensures you increase the quality of your nutrition with many essential nutrients.

You may have also been misled by mythology suggesting that protein causes cancer. This misunderstanding comes up because high-quality protein promotes the repair and growth of cells—all cells. Therefore, if a person already has cancer, excessive protein can cause those cells to grow along with every other cell in the body. Does that mean protein caused the cancer? No. As University of Illinois nutrition researcher Chris Masterjohn, PhD, notes in his review of the research related to protein and cancer, "low-protein diets depressed normal growth, increased the susceptibility to many toxins, killed toxin-exposed animals earlier, induced fatty liver, and increased the development of pre-cancerous lesions."[154] The bottom line is that eating protein causes cancer the way watering gardens causes weeds. Just as we don't effectively avoid weeds by depriving our garden of water, we don't effectively avoid cancer by depriving our body of protein. We're better served cultivating a system robust enough to ward off intruders. Fortunately, that's exactly what water-, fiber-, and protein-rich SANE foods do.

Last but not least, you may have heard the myth that protein promotes osteoporosis. This misinformation may spring from the fact that digesting protein requires more calcium than the digestion of fat or carbohydrates. Certain individuals claim this finding shows that eating a lot of protein will suck calcium from our bones—but in the case of the SANE lifestyle, these concerns are not valid.

First, as mentioned earlier, we are not eating a lot of protein—we are eating the amount humans evolved to eat. Second, with the SANE eating plan, we have no need to grab calcium from our bones, since our nonstarchy vegetable intake provides at least 150 percent more calcium than the typical US diet. (For example, leafy green vegetables are excellent sources of calcium. Calorie for calorie, spinach provides nearly twice as much calcium as reduced-fat milk.) Third, protein digestion does not negatively affect bones if intake of the mineral phosphorus is increased, and the SANE eating plan does that. Finally, while more protein increases the need for calcium, it also increases the body's ability to absorb calcium. When more protein is taken in, the body automatically makes better use of calcium. Studies show that the amount of protein we'll enjoy increases bone density by raising levels of the protein IGF-1. Researchers at Maastricht University who looked at the question of protein's impact on bones found no negative effects on net bone density or calcium status, regardless of the age of the subject. In fact, they found that dietary protein even increased bone mineral mass and reduced incidence of osteoporotic fractures in the elderly.[155]

The research is clear: Nutrient-dense protein is a critical component of long-term health and fitness.

Grocery List: Common Nutrient-Dense Proteins
(30- to 55-gram servings for a total of 100–200 grams per day)
Note: This is not an exhaustive list. The more essential nutrients packed into every calorie, the higher a protein's SANEity.

bison	hemp-protein powder	salmon
catfish	herring	sardines (and anchovies)
chicken	lamb	scallops
clams	lean conventional beef	sea bass
cod	liver	shad
cornish hen	lobster	shrimp snapper
crab	mackerel	sole
croaker	mahimahi	squid (calamari)
egg whites	mussels	swordfish
eggs	octopus	tilapia
elk	organ meats	tofu
cottage cheese	oysters	trout
plain Greek yogurt	pea-protein powder	tuna
grass-fed beef	perch	turkey
flounder	pollock	venison
haddock	pork	whey-protein powder
halibut	rabbit	whitefish
ham	rice-protein powder	

NUTRIENT-DENSE PROTEIN SUMMARY

- Nutrient-dense protein should cover a third of your plate.
- Eat protein in 30- to 55-gram servings evenly throughout the day.
- Eat a total of 100 to 200 grams of protein per day.
- Eat protein every time you eat.
- Eat seafood daily (ideally sources higher in omega-3s and lower in mercury, such as salmon, sardines, anchovies, oysters, etc.).
- High-quality, nutrient-dense sources of protein are critical.
- If you avoid animal products, you can still be SANE.

Now, let's look at the final two important aspects of the SANE eating plan: whole-food fats and low-fructose fruits.

SANE Fats and Sweets

The final step to going SANE is filling the rest of our plate with whole-food fats and low-fructose fruits.

You and I have already reviewed the research disproving that foods that contain fat are fattening, but let's put that myth to rest once and for all.

When we eat whole-food fats in place of starches and sweets, our bodies start to prefer burning fat for fuel instead of sugar. As we go SANE and get Smart about exercise, we begin to burn more calories than we're taking in—but we're not hungry and our body isn't slowing down. Why? Because it's full of nutrients and still has plenty of its preferred fuel. Sure the fuel is fat sitting on our hips instead of starch that just passed through our lips, but why would the body care? It has enough nutrition and enough energy on hand to keep us at our best.

Just the opposite happens when we regularly eat excessive starches and sweets. If we burn more calories than we're eating, our body looks around for its preferred fuel source (sugar), but doesn't find any. This deficit makes it demand more sugar and starch. We experience this as crazy carb cravings. If we're able to fight through these all-encompassing cravings and hunger pains, we've heard all about what happens next: our body burns fewer calories. But what if there's still a sugar shortage? Better burn off that sugar-hungry muscle tissue.

Still short on sugar? OK, sure, we'll eventually get to burning body fat—but why not skip the whole "feel hungry and terrible while our body cannibalizes our muscles" part and just eat delicious whole-food fat so that our body prefers to burn fat in the first place? Far from *making* us fat, eating whole-food fats instead of starches and sweets enables us to healthfully *burn* body fat.

If we set aside the myths we've been told for the past forty years, we have no reason to think that fat is bad for us. Whole foods contain fat. Whole foods were the only thing our ancestors ate for 99.8 percent of our history. How could the only foods available to us for 99.8 percent of our history harm us? If anything, we must thrive on foods that contain fats. Furthermore, the theory that fat is fattening has never been proved, despite over a billion dollars' worth of research attempting to prove it. Indeed, researchers have proved that some types of fat help burn body fat and boost health. Finally, the topper: a decline in the proportion of fat in our diet has been accompanied by the largest spike in obesity and disease rates in history.

Countless scientific studies show that worrying about eating whole-food fat is at best a distraction and at worst harmful and fattening. Research recently done at Harvard Medical School blames the decades-long emphasis on dietary fat reduction for having distracted us in the fight against the true causes of obesity. Diets high in fat have not been linked to excess body fat, either in the United States or in European countries—and, indeed, among European women, the data show that the more dietary fat women eat, the less body fat they carry. And any attempts to limit supposedly dangerous saturated fats by increasing carbohydrates just make health matters way worse—increasing triglycerides and decreasing healthy HDL cholesterol, raising glycemic load and insulin levels, and increasing the risk of diabetes and heart disease. The Harvard researchers stress that the greatest hope related to fats in the diet points not to decreasing them but to *increasing* them: "Studies and . . . trials have provided strong evidence that a higher intake of [omega-3] fatty acids from fish or plant sources lowers risk of coronary heart disease."[156]

If we want to be maximally healthy, we must eat three to six servings per day of fats contained in whole foods. When I say "whole foods," I mean foods that are not processed. All oils are processed derivatives of whole food. They contain no water, no fiber, and no protein and are therefore not substances we need to go out of our way to eat.

For example, soybean oil—whose consumption has increased about 116,300 percent over the past century—is not a whole food and actually elevates our set-point. I recommend limiting your use of oils to the small amount needed for cooking and, whenever possible, sticking with stable natural oils such as coconut oil.

But aren't we told olive oil and coconut oil are good for us? Yes, but that's relative to other oils. Think about this in the same way you thing about whole grains. Whole grains are better than refined grains, but that doesn't mean they are *good* for us. Same thing with oil: olive oil and coconut oil are much better for us than other oils (soybean, corn, vegetable, and so on), but whole olives and whole coconuts are dramatically better for us than any oil. Stable natural oils are fine for cooking, but whole foods are best for eating. (And anyone telling you to eat a tablespoon of coconut oil per day rather than eating more coconut meat may be more interested in selling you coconut oil than in your health! Everything useful that is found in coconut oil and much more is found in whole-food coconut.)

Common healthy sources of whole-food fats include seafood (salmon, sardines) and certain plants (avocado, coconut, cocoa/cacao, flax seeds, and chia seeds), unprocessed fatty cuts of meat (organic grass-fed beef), eggs, and full-fat but low-sugar dairy products (cottage cheese and plain Greek yogurt). Fatty fish, unprocessed fatty cuts of meat, eggs, and full-fat but low-sugar dairy products are one to three servings of whole-food fats depending on their size and level of fat. A serving of plant fats such as nuts and seeds is generally a small handful or three tablespoons. If the nuts are mashed into butter (natural almond butter), a serving is the size of a Ping-Pong ball, or two tablespoons.

While there are many healthy sources of whole-food fats, some are especially beneficial. We've already talked about seafood, which is one of the healthiest sources of fat in the world. Also rising to the top are cocoa/cacao, coconut, chia seeds, and milled flax seeds. As we will see later, cocoa/cacao and coconut are wonderful ways to indulge our cravings for sweets, but beyond their deliciousness, these foods are health and fat-loss powerhouses. Natural and undutched* cocoa/cacao is one of the richest

* Dutched or dutch-processed cocoa/cacao has been treated with chemicals and has lost much of its health benefit.

sources of antioxidants, polyphenols, and flavanols (hard-to-come-by healthy things) in the world. Cocoa is also packed with filling fiber and essential vitamins and nutrients. Coconut is home for a rare type of fat: medium-chain triglycerides (MCTs), which have been shown to boost metabolism. Flax seeds and chia seeds are rich sources of fiber, vitamins, and minerals, and are useful sources of omega-3 fats, extremely beneficial fats that have been shown to benefit almost every aspect of human cardiac, metabolic, and neurological health. Keep in mind that flax seeds need to be milled into a flourlike powder in order for our body to be able to make use of their abundant nutrition.

LOW-FRUCTOSE FRUITS

Much as science shows that we need to reevaluate whole-food fats, it also shows that we need to reevaluate fruits. As with every other type of food, not all fruits are created equal. Some fruits, such as berries and citrus (like oranges and grapefruit) contain healthier ratios of nutrients to sugar than common fruits such as apples, bananas, and grapes.

If you enjoy fruit, stick with one to three low-sugar fresh or frozen servings per day. A serving is roughly the size of your fist. For instance, six strawberries, one orange, half a grapefruit, or three quarters of a cup of blueberries. Focus on the fruits, such as berries and citrus, that will give you the most of what you need (nutrients) and the least of what you don't (sugar). If you can do without fruits, there is no biological reason to eat them as long as you are consuming enough nonstarchy vegetables. There's nothing essential in fruits that we cannot get, and with a lot less sugar, from nonstarchy vegetables.

Please also underline the following: fruits and vegetables are not one food group. While eating at least ten servings of nonstarchy vegetables per day will do nothing but make you healthier and slimmer, the same thing is not true for fruits, owing to their dramatically higher sugar content. Some fruits contain ten to twenty times as much sugar as some nonstarchy vegetables. For example, grapes have about nineteen times more sugar than spinach. In other words, you could eat eighteen servings of spinach and still not have eaten as much sugar as is in a single serving of grapes. Stick with zero to three servings of berries and citrus and avoid counting any fruits toward your ten servings of nonstarchy vegetables.

A SANE APPROACH TO EATING WHOLE-FOOD FATS AND LOW-FRUCTOSE FRUITS

It's helpful to enjoy whole-food fats and low-fructose fruits along with nonstarchy vegetables and nutrient-dense protein instead of on their own. For many people, eating nothing more than a cup of berries or a handful of walnuts just makes them want more berries and walnuts. This can lead to hunger, if we fight the urge, or overeating, if we give in to the urge. Eating an optimal amount of nuts and fruits is easy if we make sure they are not processed (e.g., honey-roasted nuts and fruits canned in syrup are no good) and eat them along with nonstarchy vegetables and nutrient-dense protein.

My favorite way to do this is to think of whole-food fats and low-fructose fruits as scrumptious SANE desserts. We'll cover recipes later, but the gist is that we can use nuts, nut flours, seeds, seed flours, cocoa/cacao, coconut, and berries to make SANE cookies, fudges, pies, cakes, ice cream, milkshakes, and other SANE treats that will satisfy any sweet tooth after a nonstarchy vegetable and nutrient-dense protein-rich meal.

Finally, keep in mind that if you have struggled with your weight for a long time, studies show that you are more likely to lower your set-point if you favor whole-food fats over low-fructose fruits. For example, enjoy five servings of whole-food fats per day and one serving of blueberries instead of three servings of whole-food fats, two servings of blueberries, and a handful of strawberries. As a general rule, the heavier you are, the better off you are with whole-food fats instead of low-fructose fruits. If you are extremely clogged, even the small amount of sugar in berries and citrus can slow your set-point-lowering efforts. Also, keep in mind that the less carbohydrate we eat the more fat we should eat. If you choose to live a low-carb SANE lifestyle (i.e., eating about 50 grams of carbohydrate per day), you should eat the higher-fat variants of protein.

Grocery List: Common Whole-Food Fats (3–6 servings per day)
Note: This is not an exhaustive list. The more essential nutrients provided per calorie, the more beneficial the fat.

almonds	chia seeds	kola nut	pumpkin seeds
avocado	cocoa/cacao	macadamia nuts	sesame seeds
Brazil nuts	coconut	milled flaxseed	squash seeds
cashews	hazelnuts	pecans	sunflower seeds
chestnuts	hemp seeds	pistachios	walnuts

Grocery List: Common Low-Fructose Fruits (0–3 servings per day)
Note: This is not an exhaustive list. The more essential nutrients provided per calorie, the more beneficial the fruit.

apricots	cantaloupe	honeydew melon	peaches
blackberries	casaba melon	lemon	raspberries
blueberries	cherries	lime	rhubarb
boysenberries	grapefruit	nectarine	strawberries
cranberries	guava	papaya	

WHOLE-FOOD FATS AND LOW-FRUCTOSE FRUITS SUMMARY

- Whole-food fats are essential; low-fructose fruits are not.
- Go out of your way to eat fatty seafood, cocoa/cacao, and coconut.
- Avoid unnatural processed fats (most oils) completely.
- If needed, use stable, natural processed fats such as coconut oil for cooking.
- Do away with processed fruits (canned in syrup) completely.
- Pair whole-food fats or low-fructose fruits with nonstarchy vegetables and nutrient-dense protein whenever possible.
- Whole-food fats and low-fructose fruits are SANE dessert superstars.
- If you really struggle with your weight, you will be likely to have better results if you focus on whole-food fats instead of low-fructose fruits.

In the next chapter, we'll cover ten specific tips—the Ten Principles of SANE Eating—to help us stay SANE in today's inSANE world.

The Ten Principles
of SANE Eating

PRINCIPLE 1: FREE YOURSELF
FROM CALORIE COUNTING

Anyone who recommends that we count calories is leading us down a complex and counterproductive path for three major biological reasons. First, the underpinnings of calorie counting work on the assumption that we burn a fixed number of calories every day. In other words, if we normally burn 2,000 calories per day and then cut back to eating 1,500 calories per day, it assumes that we burn 500 calories' worth of stored fat. This has been proved wrong in every study that tested it.

Second, we cannot accurately calculate how many calories we burn. The Internet is full of base metabolic rate (BMR) calculators, and gyms are filled with "cardio" machines claiming to count calories. The truth is that there is no program or tool available to nonscientists that accurately measures how many calories we burn. And even if Web-based BMR calculators and cardio-machine calculators were accurate, we would still be missing huge contributors to calories out such as:

- **Nonexercise activity thermogenesis (NEAT)**: calories burned via involuntary movement (such as fidgeting and involuntary and unnoticeable muscle movements)

- **Diet-induced thermogenesis (DIT)**: calories burned during digestion (especially when you eat protein!)
- **Muscle protein synthesis (MPS)**: calories burned in repairing lean tissue
- **Excess postexercise oxygen consumption (EPOC)**: calories burned in recovering from intense exercise

Finally, we know that fewer calories in or more calories out does not in and of itself cause the body to burn fat. Studies have shown that extremely metabolically clogged mice will burn off their vital organs as fuel and die before they burn off all their body fat for fuel. We'll never face anything this extreme, but if we starve ourselves we will become ravenously hungry, then our metabolism will slow down, then we'll burn muscle, then we'll burn fat, then we'll give in to hunger, then we'll be fatter and sicker than ever.

Our SANEr approach is to recognize that our body already balances calories and to enable it to balance us at a slimmer body composition.

PRINCIPLE 2: SHIFT FROM SHORT-TERM WEIGHT LOSS TO LONG-TERM FAT LOSS AND HEALTH

As long as we focus on short-term weight loss, our efforts will not work out long term. We need to keep this critical perspective in mind because common things that do help us lose weight short term do *not* help us stay healthy and slim long term.

The single most important step you can take to enable this mental shift is to get rid of tools that encourage starvation—e.g., your scale—and to set goals that will focus you on the long term. I know walking away from the scale is incredibly difficult. But until we free ourselves from worrying about our weight, we will risk relapsing back into our old approaches that we know do not work for the long term. Focus on getting healthier, not lighter. Your body will take care of the rest.

PRINCIPLE 3: SET MEANINGFUL GOALS AND A REALISTIC TIMETABLE

If we do not define success according to weight, then how do we define it? Swap your scale for a measuring tape.

The circumference of your waist is proved to be much more indicative of long-term wellness and aesthetics than weight. Measure your waist no more than once per month and do it on the same day of the week and at the same time to ensure the most accurate measurement possible. Alternatively, find a pair of jeans you cannot currently wear but would like to. Buy them. You will be wearing those jeans in a couple of months and, much more important, for the rest of your life. Finally, visit your doctor and have him or her measure your:

- body-fat percentage
- blood pressure
- heart rate
- fasting glucose
- triglycerides
- cholesterol

After this, pick out your top three or five goals from the list below.

- waist measurement
- body-fat percentage
- clothes test
- cholesterol level
- blood pressure
- sick less often
- mental sharpness
- sleep well
- strength
- energy level
- fitness level
- improved mood
- libido level
- confidence
- pain reduction
- athletic performance

Now file that away and don't look at it again until you've gone SANE for three months. Thanks to the misinformation we've been given, we have spent much of our entire lives creating hormonal clogs and elevating our set-point. Now we have a choice to make: Will we starve ourselves and end up worse off than we were when we started? Or, will we be patient while our body heals itself and then keeps us slim and healthy for the rest of our lives?

Healing our body in the fundamental way we're discussing here takes time. Think of it like this: You are an elite athlete who just broke your ankle. Now you have to let your body heal itself for a few months. If you follow the recommendations of top medical professionals, your body will fix itself and you will have a fully functional ankle for the rest of your life. But you need to have patience to get the best results.

Healing your metabolism is a similar process that requires a similar time line. I wish I could provide you with an exact timetable, but everyone's situation is unique. How quickly you unclog depends on many factors, including

How ambitious your goals are. More ambitious goals mean more time is needed.

How frequently and vigorously you have yo-yo dieted. More yo-yoing means more time needed.

How old you are. More years mean more time needed.

How healthy you are. More medical issues mean more time needed.

How slim your parents are. Heavier parents mean more time needed.

How you live. More stress, more alcohol, and more late nights mean more time needed.

How SANE you go. More starches and sweets means more time needed.

How should you react when you hear your friend brag about the weight she lost in a few weeks by following the latest quick-fix fad? Just smile and nod. Sadly, she will not be bragging in a few months. Her efforts are like strapping a brace around her broken ankle and going dancing. Because she is focused on the short term she has done more harm than good, but hopefully she will realize that before her body becomes even more damaged.

PRINCIPLE 4: RETHINK NUTRITION LABELS

You are already an expert in the general types of foods you can enjoy in abundance, but what about nutrition labels? How can we use them to help us identify SANE options? Here are some quick tips:

- The more fiber the better.
- The more protein the better.
- The less sugar the better.
- The fewer ingredients the better.
- The more vitamins and minerals per serving relative to calories per serving the better.
- If the ingredients include added sweeteners that contain calories (see the list provided earlier), hydrogenated anything, trans anything, starch (flour, corn, rice, barley, etc.), or anything you cannot pronounce, avoid it.
- Don't pay too much attention to percentages. They do not reflect the actual Nutrition—nutrients per calorie—of the food. For example, it's easy to be led to believe that a "low-calorie" serving of sugar-saturated cereal is "healthy" because it provides 25 percent of the of vitamin C necessary to avoid malnutrition. That's incorrect.
- Don't pay attention to labels at all, since the most SANE foods available (nonstarchy vegetables, seafood, meat, raw nuts and seeds, low-fructose fruits, and so on) frequently don't have nutrition labels on them. You could even imagine that a major reason why we have nutrition labels at all is that much of what we find at the grocery store these days is so far from food that we have no way of knowing its health value without explicit instructions.

PRINCIPLE 5: SAVE MONEY— BUY GROCERIES IN BULK

You can cut the cost of going SANE in half if you do your grocery shopping at bulk wholesalers like Costco and Sam's Club or at farmers' markets. If you do not have access to these options, then buy enough nonstarchy vegetables and nutrient-dense protein at your conventional grocery store to last you until they go on sale again. Frozen and freezable options are key in this scenario.

PRINCIPLE 6: MASTER SNACKING AND ON-THE-GO EATING

You will find that you won't need to snack much because your meals will be full of Satisfying food. As a general rule, if you need to snack, you're probably not eating enough SANE foods at mealtimes and should reassess the composition of those meals. But if you need a little energy boost or you're simply craving a sweet, salty, or crunchy treat, here are my top ten go-to options:

Top 10 SANE Snacks and Treats

1. hard- or soft-boiled eggs (tip: add half a teaspoon of baking soda per quart of boiling water and cool the eggs in ice water after boiling to make peeling easy)
2. raw nonstarchy vegetables with guacamole
3. SANE smoothies (see recipes on page 223)
4. low-sugar jerky or unprocessed lunch meats
5. protein bars (make sure they contain at least five times more protein than sugar—I recommend Quest bars, which have a greater than 10:1 ratio of protein to sugar, are made from quality ingredients, and are high in fiber)
6. berries and/or low-sugar protein powder mixed with plain Greek yogurt or cottage cheese
7. SANE treats, like fudge, cake, pie, cookies, pudding, or ice cream (see recipes on page 236)
8. baked kale chips
9. nuts or seeds
10. sugar-free drinks with as few chemicals in them as possible (ideally these would be sweetened with a natural noncaloric sweetener such as stevia)

These options can also come in handy while you're traveling. Also note that freezing food, putting it in an insulated bag, and enjoying it after it thaws is another useful option. If you are eating out, avoid pasta dishes, and ask your server to "hold the starch, double the vegetables." Asian restaurants are easy: eat the whole main dish and skip the rice instead of eating half of the main dish and a bunch of rice. If burgers are your only option, get a gigantic grass-fed or lean one and enjoy it without the bun.

PRINCIPLE 7: SIMPLIFY WITH GREEN SMOOTHIES

While blending is not required, eating ten or more servings of nonstarchy vegetables per day is much easier if you use a good blender to make nonstarchy vegetable and low-fructose fruit smoothies. Don't use a juicer. It removes fiber and healthy nutrients. Use a blender and customize this general formula:

1. Pack as much spinach as you can into a good blender (Vitamix and Blendtec are excellent; Ninjas are quite good and less expensive).
2. Add one or two handfuls of fresh or frozen strawberries or an orange (optional: along with some of the natural noncaloric sweetener stevia or xylitol).
3. Add 30 grams of vanilla-flavored low-sugar protein powder and a little cinnamon.
4. Add water and ice cubes.
5. Blend completely.
6. Adjust the amount of low-sugar fruit, cinnamon, water, and ice cubes to make your perfect green smoothie.

The neat thing about these smoothies is that by following these instructions, you will be able to consume two to five servings of nonstarchy vegetables raw while drinking something that tastes like a strawberry or orange Creamsicle. It's hard to believe until you try it, but the taste of the spinach is completely masked by the low-fructose fruits and vanilla. And talk about convenience. You can make a few of these at a time, enjoy them on the go throughout the day, and take care of your nonstarchy vegetable goal without having to cook.

As you get more advanced with your green smoothies, you will find nonstarchy vegetable combinations that will provide you with more nutrition in a quick and portable smoothie than most people consume in a week. Green smoothies may seem scary at first, but after trying them for a week and seeing how you look and feel, you may find that living without them starts to feel even scarier.

PRINCIPLE 8: PROTECT YOUR SANEity AT EVENTS AND HOLIDAYS

Starches and sweets are everywhere during the holidays. The key to preserving your SANEity is going to sound familiar: keep yourself so satisfied with water-, fiber-, and protein-rich foods that you are too full for these sugar bombs—or at least so you can enjoy a bite and walk away smiling. If you know you are about to step into a starch- and sweet-saturated situation, then eat a lot of nonstarchy vegetables, nutrient-dense protein, and whole-food fats *before* you get to the party or walk into the lounge.

Of course, it's fine to splurge occasionally, especially when we splurge intelligently by focusing on fatty rather than sugary or starchy treats. If you have to pick something from the cheese and meat platter or the cookie platter, splurge on the fatty cheeses and meats. Natural fats are a wonderful treat because they fill us up while keeping our fat-storing hormones at bay. Sugary starches do just the opposite. Splurge on fat to avoid storing fat.

Finally, many of these situations actually make staying clog-free simple, as buffets offer an array of nonstarchy vegetables, fruits, cheeses, meats, seafood, nuts, starches, and sweets. Fill half your plate up with nonstarchy vegetables; fill most of the other half with seafood and meat; fill in the gap with low-fructose fruits, nuts, and cheeses; and enjoy. Still hungry? Repeat the first plate. As we know, the key to long-term success isn't avoiding food. Hunger is unhealthy.

PRINCIPLE 9: ENJOY LOTS OF WATER AND GREEN TEA

Your body requires at least eight glasses of water per day to burn body fat effectively. More is better. Drinking a lot of water decreases the concentration of various substances in our blood, and this increases our body's ability to burn fat (this is called hypo-osmolality). Additionally, continuously drinking cold water raises our metabolic rate. Studies show we burn about two additional calories for every ounce of cold water we drink.

If your urine is not clear, if you are ever thirsty, or if you have room to drink things other than water—or green tea—then you could be slimmer and healthier by drinking more water.

The easiest way to drink an optimal amount of water is to fill up a gallon (128-ounce) jug in the morning and to make sure it is empty two hours before you go to bed. Another great way to boost your water intake is to fall in love with green tea.

Green tea comes from the same plant as black tea (the tea most common in the United States and Europe) but it is processed differently. Its unique processing leaves green tea with a large amount of substances called polyphenols—especially EGCG (epigallocatechin gallate). From a health perspective, the polyphenols in green tea have been shown to help prevent:

weight gain	Alzheimer's disease
cancer	kidney stones
hypertension	eye issues
cardiovascular disease	atherosclerosis
dental issues	low-HDL cholesterol
insulin resistance	inflammatory bowel disease
virus infections	diabetes
bone issues	liver disease
Parkinson's disease	bacterial issues

The body fat burned by green tea well outweighs the body-fat-burning effects of the small amount of caffeine in it (which is one-fifth the caffeine in a cup of coffee). Researchers suspect green tea's unique fat-burning effect has to do with the interaction of this tea's polyphenols, caffeine, and the hormone noradrenaline. To maximize all the benefits green tea has to offer, aim to drink ten bags' worth of it per day.

Now you may be thinking, "Ten bags of green tea on top of all that water? I'm going to spend all day in the bathroom, I'll be really jittery, and I won't have any money left. Isn't that too much fluid, too much caffeine, and too much money?" Not if we're smart about it:

HYDRATION: All the green tea we drink counts toward our water goals. If you drink ten eight-ounce cups of green tea, that counts as ten eight-ounce cups of water. Also, you can brew a lot of green tea in a little water. For example, I brew eight bags of green tea at a time in eight ounces of water. I let it sit for a few minutes, add ice, and then drink it quickly. Do that once in the morning and once in the afternoon and you are good to go.

CAFFEINE: Decaf green tea is as healthy and helpful as regular green tea.

You can choose decaffeinated green tea and get the same health benefits, but if you crave caffeine like me, never fear: a bag of regular green tea contains only about 30 milligrams of caffeine. Compare that with a cup of brewed coffee, which can contain up to 150 milligrams of caffeine. Most doctors will advise that up to 300 milligrams of caffeine per day (the equivalent of two cups of coffee) is safe. Ten bags of green tea deliver roughly the same amount of caffeine to your body as two cups of coffee.

8 oz (Unless Otherwise Noted)	Caffeine (mg)
1 max-strength NoDoz pill	200
brewed coffee	150
1 bag black tea	80
Monster energy drink	80
Rockstar energy drink	80
1.5 ounces espresso	77
Red Bull energy drink	76
Full Throttle energy drink	72
1 bag green tea	30
decaffeinated coffee	7
1 bag decaf green tea	3

COST-EFFECTIVENESS: It is cheap and easy to buy regular or decaf green tea in bulk. I buy it online in bulk each month and the cost comes to $0.08 per bag—including shipping and handling. That is less than a dollar a day to get all the benefits green tea has to offer.

Also keep in mind that there is a big difference between drinking tea for enjoyment and drinking green tea for health. Tea is like wine. Just as there is $5 wine and $500 wine, there is $0.08 green tea and $8.00 green tea. If you already enjoy more expensive tea, keep it up and add drinking at least ten bags of less expensive green tea to your day.

If you don't enjoy hot tea, add ice and drink it cold. If you prefer not to drink caffeine, try decaf. If you don't want to stain your teeth, drink it through a straw. If you don't like the taste, drink it with something SANE you do like, such as a green smoothie. And stick to sipping green tea instead of swallowing green tea supplements. Studies show that most green tea supplements are not as good for us as natural green tea.

If you are interested in optimizing green tea's health benefits, studies suggest that you would be best served blending matcha green tea with a peeled lemon and water for two minutes (or until the lemon is completely liquefied).

Finally, drinking more water and green tea makes it easier to avoid sugary beverages. If it is not water, green tea, or something else calorie free—e.g., coffee without cream or sugar—or something you personally blended from SANE foods, drinking it will raise your set-point fast and furiously.

PRINCIPLE 10: FORGET PERFECTION. COMMIT PUBLICLY. GET SUPPORT.

It is reasonable to reach this point and say, "I can't do all of that" or "I don't want to do all of that." No problem. This isn't about being perfect. In fact, pursuing nutritional perfection is stressful, is bad for your health, and is called orthorexia (*orthos* = correct or right, *orexis* = appetite). Avoid becoming orthorexic. Focus on getting the big things right most of the time. Arm yourself with the information necessary to look and feel good and apply as much or as little of it as you like depending on how much body fat you want to lose and how much better you want to feel.

What most people find is that they start doing the basics outlined here, love the results, and then want to go further. Again, SANE eating favors practicality over perfection and you can burn as little or as much body fat as you want to. Want to burn up to two pounds of body fat per week? Eat so much SANE food that you are too full for inSANE food and exercise smarter. Have more modest goals? Eat less SANE food and some inSANE food. You make the decision. The more nonstarchy vegetables and nutrient-dense protein you eat, the slimmer you will be.

The table below details a spectrum of eating and lifestyle choices, and gives you an indication of the results for each set of behaviors. Take a brief look and identify where you fit on this spectrum currently, and where you would like to end up. Please note that this and everything else like it are general guides. I urge you not to get bogged down in details, as slim really is simple once we have access to the correct information. Eat so many nonstarchy vegetables and nutrient-dense proteins that you are too full for starches and sweets, exercise smarter for a few minutes per week, give your body a few months to heal itself, and you will achieve a previously unimaginable level of *lasting* slimness and health.

HOW FOOD AND LIFESTYLE CHOICES ADD UP

A Formula for Obesity

- Avoid eating nutrient-dense protein.
- Eat mostly starch and sweets.
- Eat inSANE desserts all the time.
- Drink anything other than water or green tea.

Which amounts to eating this daily:

>12 servings of starch or sweets

0 servings of nutrient-dense protein

0 servings of nonstarchy vegetables

0 servings of whole-food fats

0 servings of low-fructose fruits

0 ounces of water / 0 bags of green tea

Get less than six hours of undisturbed sleep per night.

A Formula for Being Overweight

- Eat at least 30 grams of nutrient-dense protein with lunch or dinner.
- Trade starch and sweets for nutrient-dense protein and nonstarchy vegetables at most dinners.
- Eat inSANE desserts sometimes and SANE desserts at other times.
- Drink water and green tea occasionally.

Which amounts to eating this daily:

9 servings of starch or sweets

One 30- to 55-gram serving of nutrient-dense protein

2 servings of nonstarchy vegetables

1 serving of whole-food fats
0–1 serving of low-fructose fruits
32 ounces of water / 2 bags of green tea

	Get six hours of undisturbed sleep per night.
A Formula for Being Typical	• Eat at least 30 grams of nutrient-dense protein with lunch and dinner. • Trade starch and sweets for nutrient-dense protein and nonstarchy vegetables at lunch and dinner. • Eat an inSANE dessert once per week, and SANE desserts a couple of times per week. • Actively try to drink more water and green tea.

Which amounts to eating this daily:
6 servings of starch or sweets
Two 30- to 55-gram servings of nutrient-dense protein
5 servings of nonstarchy vegetables
2 servings of whole-food fats
0–2 servings of low-fructose fruits
64 ounces of water / 5 bags of green tea
Get seven hours of undisturbed sleep per night.

A Formula for Being Fit	• Eat at least 30 grams of nutrient-dense protein with breakfast, lunch, and dinner. • Almost always trade starch and sweets for protein and nonstarchy vegetables. • Eat SANE desserts a couple of times per week. • Drink water and green tea often.

Which amounts to eating this daily:
3 servings of starch or sweets
Three 30- to 55-gram servings of nutrient-dense protein
8 servings of nonstarchy vegetables
3 servings of whole-food fats
0–3 servings of low-fructose fruits
96 ounces of water / 8 bags of green tea

Get eight hours of undisturbed sleep per night and exercise smarter.

A Formula for Being a Fitness Model	• Eat at least 30 grams of nutrient-dense protein with at least breakfast, lunch, and dinner.
	• Always trade starch and sweets for nutrient-dense protein and nonstarchy vegetables.
	• Eat SANE desserts occasionally, not because you are depriving yourself, but because you are often too full for dessert.
	• Drink so much water and green tea that you don't have room to drink anything other than unsweetened coffee.

| *Which amounts to eating this daily:* |
| 0 servings of starch or sweets |
| Three to six 30- to 55-gram servings of nutrient-dense protein (100–200 grams total) |
| >10 servings of nonstarchy vegetables |
| 3–6 servings of whole-food fats |
| 0–3 servings of low-fructose fruit |
| 128 ounces water / 10+ bags of green tea |

| Get eight or more hours of undisturbed sleep per night and exercise smarter. |

Regardless of your individual goals, commit to them. Publicly, if possible. E-mail those goals to family and friends. Post them on your social networks and in this book's online support group (www.SANE Solution.com). Draw support and motivation from those who love you and others who are enjoying a similar lifestyle.

When people ask you how much weight you have lost, tell them you have no idea, but you are wearing jeans you couldn't zip up three months ago, have an absurd amount of energy, are falling asleep the minute your head hits the pillow, are free from medical conditions previously plaguing you, and are playing as much tennis as you did in high school. You will not be bragging. You will be setting an example of what health and fitness success really means, and you may change their lives while changing your own.

Now that we've covered how to go SANE with your food choices, we're going to look at how you can get Smarter with your exercise routine—

and it takes only about twenty minutes a week. A little smarter exercise clears hormonal clogs more effectively than a lot of traditional exercise thanks to its high potency. Let's look at how to make it work for you.

From Pastry Chef to SANE Gourmet: Carrie's Story

Carrie started her career as one of the best pastry chefs in England. She also started her life as a naturally thin person. She could enjoy all the inSANE treats she liked while staying slim and without even thinking about joining a gym.

Then she hit her late thirties. Nothing about her lifestyle changed, but her body did. She watched in horror as the same body that had automatically kept her slim for over three decades became her enemy.

> Now I know that just like everyone else's, my hormones and set-point were changing with age. But, I had no idea about this at the time and got depressed. My worst moment involved a trip to the doctor.
>
> I visited my doctor to get help with my weight issues. My doctor told me to drink only weight-loss shakes and exercise as much as possible for two weeks. He said this would prove that I could control my weight. What followed were two horrible weeks. I was able to "find" 15 hours per week to exercise, but they came at the expense of relationships and my career. I was constantly hungry, tired, and in a mental fog. You can imagine the impact on my personal and professional life. But, doctors know best.
>
> After two weeks of misery, I went back to my doctor and hit an all-time low when I found out my weight hadn't changed at all. I fired my doctor and started to look for alternatives.
>
> SANE eating appealed to me because it was diverse enough that I could continue to make delicious dishes, and it was food friendly enough that I could swear off hunger forever. Smarter exercise was a no-brainer, as anything more than 30 minutes of exercise per week simply doesn't work with my schedule.
>
> In just a few months I was back to my slim self despite having crossed the 40-year mark. I'm still creating culinary treats with simple SANE substitutions. I'm never hungry. My friends have no idea how I

eat so much, exercise so little, and stay so slim. My LDL cholesterol also fell 100 points.

I'm now dedicating a large part of my life to sharing delicious SANE dishes with everyone I can. I know firsthand that eating lots of delicious food and being healthy and slim doesn't have to be an either/or decision. I know that not eating and doing a lot of exercise "works" for some people, but I'm not one of them.

Get Smart with Your Exercise

Traditional exercise programs require a commitment of at least ten hours per week. This requirement alone accounts for much of their long-term failure rate (which is around 95 percent). Who has that much spare time?

Fortunately, scientists have discovered a smarter alternative. A safer and more potent form of exercise that unclogs us in just ten to twenty minutes per week. How can it possibly do so much in so little time? "Smarter" exercise, as I like to call it, does something much different from traditional exercise. It exercises *all* our muscle fibers, including a type of muscle fiber that is especially hormonally helpful and has probably never been activated in your entire life! Contrast this with traditional exercise that activates only the one least hormonally helpful type of muscle fiber. By working additional and more powerful muscle fibers we can exercise less—but smarter—and create a set-point-lowering response that is impossible via any traditional exercise.

Let's quickly compare traditional exercise with this smarter alternative. Traditional exercise is rooted in the false calorie-counting theory. It aims to burn calories and is done frequently, for a long time; uses a little resistance; and often leads to injury (think jogging.) On the other hand, smarter exercise is rooted in proven physiology. It aims to clear our hormonal clog and is done less frequently, for a short period of time; uses a lot of resistance; and is extremely safe. Smarter exercise is done as eccentric resistance training and no-impact interval training, and it's one of the most exciting things I have to share with you.

Not only does exercising smarter give you all the benefits that traditional exercise programs claim to provide, but it is also the only activity that has been proved to reverse aging in humans at the molecular level. Scientists at the Buck Institute for Age Research discovered that after six months of resistance training "the transcriptional signature of aging was markedly reversed back to that of younger levels for most genes that were affected by both age and exercise." [157] Presented with the findings from this study, Dr. Doug McGuff, author of *Body by Science*, remarked, "Nothing else in human history has shown a functional reversing of age in humans at a molecular level." [158]

Best of all, smarter exercise is simple. You'll notice as you read this section that I spend a lot less time talking about exercise than I do covering nutrition. That's not because I don't value the role of exercise in a healthy lifestyle, but because exercising for long-term health and fat loss has been overcomplicated and SANE eating accounts for at least 90 percent of our long-term success. As author Tim Caulfield brilliantly states, "When you hear someone say 'I work out so I can eat what I want,' you should know that he is deluded unless (a) he is training as hard as a Tour de France cyclist but doesn't care about his weight; or (b) 'eat what I want' means the unbridled consumption of broccoli, celery, water, and air." [159]

Smarter exercise is a wonderful and required complement to a SANE lifestyle, but much the way exercise cannot undo the damage done to our respiratory system by smoking, the same is true for the damage done to our metabolic system by inSANE foods. By focusing primarily on eating more but smarter, and secondarily on exercising less but smarter, you can simplify your life while enjoying long-term results you never thought possible.

WILL SMARTER EXERCISE MAKE ME BIGGER?

Before we change our minds, bodies, and genes long term with the Six Principles of Smarter Exercise, let's address the common fear that using weight-resistance-based exercise makes women look like men and men look like bulldogs. The best way to address this fear is to understand our biology.

The levels of testosterone needed to develop bulky muscles are found in only a small percentage of men. Most women have about the same level of testosterone as a ten-year-old boy. We all also have a gene called GDF-8, and it controls a substance called myostatin, which further regulates the amount of muscle we have and how much it develops naturally. The base levels of hormones, myostatin, and muscle in nearly all women and most men make it impossible for them to naturally build bulky muscles using any form of exercise.

Think of muscle size as being like muscle speed. Few people are fast because few people have "fast-muscle genes." No matter how much most people run, they will never get faster than their genes allow. However, if people do have the genes for speed, they will naturally be faster than most people without ever training.

Similarly, few people can become bulky because few people—particularly women—have "bulky-muscle genes." No matter how much resistance training most people do, they will never develop more muscle than their genes allow them to. As William Kraemer, PhD, the editor of the *Journal of Strength and Conditioning Research*, tells us, "Women have been sold a myth of becoming big. They do not have the genetics."[160]

Also keep in mind that body fat is bulky, not muscle. This is why some trainers will tell you, "Muscle weighs more than body fat." While muscle does not weigh more than body fat—one pound of muscle weighs the same as one pound of fat, which weighs the same as one pound of feathers—muscle does take up less space. This is why most female fitness models are about five feet six inches and weigh 140 pounds. We look at them, and judging by their size, think they weigh 110 pounds. They do not. See those toned legs? That is quite a bit of muscle tissue taking up a little space.

Far from causing a problem, developing compact muscle tissue via smarter exercise is one of our most effective tools to boost health and burn body fat *long term*. In fact, Yasuhiro Izumiya, MD, PhD, a molecular cardiologist at Boston University, found that development of the specific type of muscle fibers targeted by smarter exercise "can regress obesity and resolve metabolic disorders in obese mice."[161] Notably, Izumiya doesn't mention "burning calories" or "working up a sweat," but rather mentions "resolving metabolic disorders." The latter is all about the long term. All those other things focus on the short term.

Izumiya went on to describe how these muscle fibers cleared clogs by improving "insulin sensitivity and [causing] reductions in blood glucose, insulin, and leptin levels." Most encouragingly, he noted, "These effects occurred despite a *reduction* in physical activity."

We will get more for less, and we will see that far from being too good to be true, once we understand our physiology, smarter exercise is too obvious to be false.

Laying the "Exercise to Burn Calories" Myth to Rest Once and for All

Freeing ourselves from thinking about exercise in terms of calories isn't easy after a lifetime of incorrect information. However, it becomes easier once we learn how traditional exercise is terrible at burning calories. Thirty minutes of jogging consumes only 170 more calories than we would have burned spending thirty minutes with our family and friends.

To put 170 calories into perspective, our liver burns over three times that amount per day. In other words, we would have to do ninety minutes of conventional cardiovascular exercise every day to burn as many calories as our liver does every day. Three-quarters of the calories we burn every day have nothing to do with moving, let alone traditional aerobic exercise.

In fact, remember the guideline "eat three to six 30- to 55-gram servings of protein per day to activate muscle protein synthesis" in our earlier discussion? Researchers at the University of Illinois have found that when we eat a SANE quantity and quality of protein, we can trigger the creation of about 250 grams of new tissue within our body per day. This process can cost a whopping 30 percent of the total calories we burn in a day (about 540 to 720 calories). It is so calorically costly, that it causes our cells to generate more mitochondria (metabolic power plants)—a reaction once thought possible only via intense exercise. I bring this up because it shows that even if our goal was to burn calories, eating a SANE quantity and quality of protein would cause our body to burn more calories than any normal person would ever burn via aerobic exercise.

As we will cover shortly, being active is wonderful for our health. We should do as much low-impact restorative activity such as walking, yoga, etc., as possible. However, even if we fell back into the calorie myths, traditional aerobic exercises such as jogging still wouldn't effectively further those misdirected goals. As Eric Oliver, PhD, at the University of Chicago tells us, "For Americans to begin losing weight through [traditional cardiovascular] exercise, the current USDA exercise guideline would have to be increased by almost 200 percent. . . . Americans would need to start exercising at least two hours a day, six days a week."[162]

Forget calories. Focus on hormones. Lower your set-point. Burn body fat forever.

The Six Principles
of Smarter Exercise

Gradually, weight lifting [resistance training] changed the way I looked. The alteration was not dramatic, but I loved it. My back became broader, which makes my hips look smaller; my arms and legs are firmer and more shapely. I never grew big muscles, but they are defined; you can see their outlines. I feel different, too, more confident of my body's strength and of my ability to do almost any movement in daily life with little effort.

—Gina Kolata, *New York Times*[163]

PRINCIPLE 1: EXERCISE MORE
MUSCLE TO GET MORE RESULTS

Why do people ride a bike to burn body fat instead of drawing pictures of bikes to burn body fat? After all, both activities exercise muscles. We choose to ride a bike because doing so exercises more muscle (the large leg muscles) than drawing bikes (the small hand muscles). The more muscle exercised, the better our results. Traditional exercise has that much right. However, we can do a lot better.

Just as we get better results in less time by working more muscles within our body, we get even better results in even less time by concentrating our efforts on exercising more of the the individual fibers that make up our muscles. Boston University researchers found that when we engage in exercise that works more muscle fibers, we exercise the uniquely clog-clearing muscle fibers called type 2b muscle fibers, which have "a previously unappreciated role in regulating whole-body metabolism [unclogging]."[164] Because of that role, the researchers concluded that strength training might be even more important to overweight people.

So how do we activate these and all the rest of our muscle fibers? The answer may surprise you. The best strategy is to exercise *less*—but smarter. Here's how this works. Just as we have different muscles to do different things—our biceps help move our arms and our hamstrings help move our legs—we also have different muscle fibers to perform different roles within the tissue that makes up our muscles. For instance, the type 1 (slow-twitch) fibers in our arms, our legs, and every other muscle group enable us to move with a little force for hours. They keep us walking around all day. On the other hand, type 2 (fast-twitch) fibers enable us to move with a lot of force for minutes and seconds. They enable us to lift furniture briefly and they come in three forms: type 2a, type 2x, and type 2b—each getting progressively stronger, larger, and hormonally helpful (I'll dig into hormones in a minute).

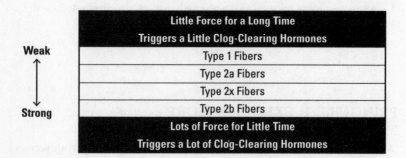

Just as our stronger, larger leg muscles help us burn more fat than our smaller, weaker hand muscles, our stronger, larger type 2 fibers help us burn more fat than our weaker type 1 fibers. Similarly, much as we engage more muscle groups when we lift a heavy object (we lift heavy boxes with our legs, back, and arms, while we lift light boxes with only our arms), we also use more muscle fibers the heavier the object we move (we use type 1 and all type 2 fibers when we do smarter exercise, while we use only our type 1 fibers when we jog).

When we put all of this together, we arrive at a surprising and encouraging conclusion. The more resistance we use, the more muscle fibers we work, the more energy we use, the faster we run out of energy, the more sore we get, and therefore, the less exercise we need to do in terms of both duration (exercise for about ten minutes at a time) and frequency (once or twice per week) to burn fat and boost our health long term. For instance, we can't hold a heavy box (a lot of muscle fibers worked) as long or as often as we can hold a light box (a few fibers worked).

Hormonal Healing Potential	Worked via Less, Smarter Exercise	Worked via More, Traditional Exercise
Type 1 Muscle Fibers	✓	✓
Type 2a Muscle Fibers	✓	
Type 2x Muscle Fibers	✓	
Type 2b Muscle Fibers	✓	

This means the choice between exercising more, but with less resistance, and exercising less, but with more resistance, is clear. If we choose to follow the traditional guidance and to exercise more, we have to pick an exercise that requires a little force, engages few muscle fibers, and requires a little energy. We then do this exercise for a long time before we run out of energy and we get little hormonal benefit. Further, it does not make us particularly sore so we are compelled to do it frequently. However, if we choose to exercise smarter—i.e., with more resistance—we pick an exercise that requires a lot of force, many muscle fibers, and a lot of energy. We then run out of energy in a short time and we achieve dramatic hormonal benefits. We also get quite sore and are unable to do it frequently. In short, we get more results in less time. As Dr. Ralph Carpinelli, of the Human Performance Laboratory at Adelphi University, clearly states, "There is little scientific evidence, and no theoretical physiological basis, to suggest that a greater volume of exercise elicits greater increases in strength or hypertrophy [muscle development]."[165]

Is this strategy a way of cutting corners? I don't think so. When we think about the class genius who aces her test in half the time it takes others to get a C, we don't say she's cutting corners. We call her *smart*.

So why do many other programs suggest that we work fewer muscle fibers for a longer periods of time (via conventional cardio)? For the same reasons so many diet programs suggest starving ourselves: They are rooted in the calorie myths. They are focused on mythical metabolism math and manually burning more calories. They fight against our set-point and therefore rarely work long term.

Finally, it's important to note that exercising with more resistance doesn't mean that you have to put more stress on your joints. The techniques that follow will allow you to increase resistance and maximize the results of your workout without increasing the impact on your body. These exercises are safer than the high-impact cardio activities many people embrace, such as running. So let's focus on increasing your results while decreasing the amount of time you spend at the gym.

PRINCIPLE 2: FOCUS ON HORMONES INSTEAD OF CALORIES

Traditional exercise is all about "burning calories." In case you haven't noticed, research reveals traditional exercise is all wrong.

Smarter exercise ignores the quantity of calories burned during the 1 percent of your life spent exercising. It focuses on how you exercise, which is to say what muscle fibers you engage, and on triggering more clog-clearing hormones. All you need to harness these hormones is to apply the first principle: exercise with more resistance to work more muscle to get more results.

Why should we focus on hormones instead of calories when exercising? One of the reasons our body slows down and burns muscle before it burns body fat is that burning body fat is hard. Until we get the right combination of hormones, we are not burning through anything meaningful other than time and muscle tissue. The other reason is that our body does not want to burn fat unless it has no other option. It is unfortunate for our waistlines, but it makes perfect survival sense. Our body stores fat to protect us from starving. If it burns fat, it cannot protect us.

"Hard to do" plus "do not want to do" generally equals "it's not happening." That is, unless our body has no other option. The way to achieve this is simple: require it to expend a huge amount of energy quickly. Use more resistance. Exercise smarter. Work all muscle fibers.

As we know, when our body needs a lot of energy it can do four things: Make us eat more. Slow down. Burn muscle. Burn fat. However, when we exercise with a lot of resistance, we eliminate three of these options. Making us eat more will not work because digestion takes a long time. It is too late to slow us down because the energy demands have already been made. Burning muscle is out of the question, since smarter exercise stimulates muscle rather than destroying it. Left with no other option, our body is forced to produce hormones such as epinephrine, adrenaline, noradrenaline, growth hormone, etc., which free up energy stored as body fat.

Please keep in mind that increasing the frequency or duration of exercise does not yield the same results as increasing the resistance of our exercise. More frequent or longer workouts are akin to a martial artist trying to break four progressively thicker boards by gently tapping on them more. Breaking through the boards is about higher quality (force), not higher quantity (duration and frequency). With one focused, quick, safe, and intense strike, the martial artist will achieve something no quantity of lower quality could ever accomplish. Similarly, with one focused, quick, safe, and intense workout, we will achieve something no quantity of lower quality ever could. We will break—in a healthy way— each of our progressively stronger types of muscle fibers and achieve a set-point-lowering reaction no quantity of lower quality ever could.

PRINCIPLE 3: INCREASE RESISTANCE AND REDUCE FREQUENCY TO INCREASE RESULTS

If we have more hair cut off when we get a haircut, we can get haircuts less often. That is not some too-good-to-be-true gimmick. That is common sense. The more hair we have cut off, the more time needed to grow it back. Similarly, if we exercise more muscle, we can exercise less often, because more time is required to recover.

How long our muscles take to recover is a great way to tell if we are exercising smarter. If we are able to exercise on Monday and then do the same thing a day or two later, we are not activating all our muscle fibers. If Monday's workout used enough resistance to exercise all our muscle fibers, they will not be ready to go again one, two, three, four, or even five days later. Type 2b muscle fibers need at least six days to recover.

If we are exercising frequently, either we are not exercising smarter or we are not giving our clog-clearing hormones enough time to do their job. Either way we are spending more time exercising and burning less body fat long term. Enough of that. Let's do a little smarter exercise and then let our unclogged bodies do the rest.

PRINCIPLE 4: LOWER WEIGHTS TO LOWER YOUR WEIGHT

Smarter exercise does not require lifting weights. We are going to focus on lowering weights.

Every resistance training exercise has two parts: lifting the resistance (for example, standing up) and lowering the resistance (for example, sitting down). Lifting the resistance is called the *concentric* portion of the exercise. Concentric is when the muscle contracts. Lowering the resistance is called the *eccentric* portion of the exercise. Eccentric is when the muscle extends. Lifting weights—the concentric action—gets more attention in muscle magazines. But lowering weights—the eccentric action—gets more results in studies.

While lifting weights helps boys feel like men, safely and slowly lowering weights enables us to use up to 40 percent more resistance. That enables more muscle fibers to be worked and more clog-clearing hormones to be triggered. That means more results in less time. For example, Marc Roig, PhD, of the Department of Physical Therapy at the University of British Columbia, found that "eccentric training performed at high intensities was shown to be more effective in promoting increases in muscle."[166]

Focusing on the eccentric—lowering—portion of resistance training works so well because it safely allows our muscles to generate more force. To test this principle, walk up a flight of stairs and then walk back down them. Notice how the trip down was easier? That is because your muscles are stronger while doing eccentric—lowering—actions on the way down. Or if you want to take this test one step further and eliminate the influence of gravity, hop onto a seated row or chest press machine (or any exercise that moves horizontally), and select a weight that you cannot lift with one arm but can lift easily with two arms. Lift it with two arms and cautiously relax one arm and observe how you are able to lower the resistance with one arm. You couldn't lift the weight with one arm, but you could lower it with one arm because, as Neil Reeves, PhD, of Manchester Metropolitan University, tells us, "Muscles are capable of developing much higher forces when they contract eccentrically compared with when they contract concentrically."[167]

Once we understand this principle, we can see why it is less effective to focus on lifting resistance. It's a bit like writing with our nondominant hand. It "works," but we know how our body operates best, so why not leverage that to do better work in less time? We'll cover how in part 3.

PRINCIPLE 5: REDUCE TIME EXERCISING TO REDUCE BODY FAT

> This novel time-efficient training paradigm can be used as a strategy to reduce metabolic risk factors in young and middle-aged sedentary populations who otherwise would not adhere to time-consuming traditional aerobic exercise regimes.
>
> —Dr. John Babraj, Heriot-Watt University[168]

As we covered earlier, the more muscle we exercise, the more energy we use and the less exercise we can do. This point is extremely important and is worth rephrasing and repeating because all we ever hear is "exercise more."

We have a limited amount of energy. If exercise Y takes five minutes to use up our energy but exercise X takes an hour to use up our energy, then exercise Y uses much more muscle and is much more metabolically beneficial than exercise X. We will be doing smarter exercise for just a few minutes per week because it's physically impossible to do a lot of smarter exercise. We run out of energy and the body shuts down, whether we like it or not.

The best way to exercise smarter is the eccentric training that we just covered and will dig deeper into momentarily. However, if you enjoy using cardio machines such as stationary bikes or ellipticals to exercise, you can do those smarter—using more resistance—as well. Let's call this smarter interval training. Experts at Pennington Biomedical Research Center have found that interval training stimulates the body to improve insulin sensitivity more than low-quality/high-quantity cardiovascular exercise. In order to tap into that smarter cardio response, we have to update the way we think about cardiovascular exercises.[169]

Contrary to popular belief, cardiovascular exercises and resistance training exercises are not completely different. Traditional cardiovascular exercises are resistance-training exercises that require little force and work only our weakest muscle fibers.

Say we get on a leg-press resistance-training machine, add no resistance, and move our legs up and down for thirty minutes. Did we do resistance training or cardiovascular exercise? Our hormones don't care. Our muscles did not have to generate much force, so we did nothing to lower our set-point. Or say we get on a stair-stepper cardiovascular exercise machine, add no resistance, and move our legs up and down for thirty minutes. Did we do resistance training or cardiovascular exercise? Our muscles don't care.

Now let's say we get on a stationary bike, increase the resistance so much that the only way we can generate enough force to move the pedals is to stand up as we pedal. Let's say we then pedal as hard as we can for thirty seconds, at which point we have to stop because we are out of energy. Did we do

1. Resistance training?
2. Cardiovascular exercise?
3. Neither?
4. Both?
5. It does not matter—our muscles had to generate a lot of force and therefore we triggered the hormonal reaction we're after?

Answer: *5—IT DOES NOT MATTER.* Our body does not care about resistance training or cardiovascular training. It responds in terms of how many muscle fibers an exercise works. So the question then becomes: "How do we use more muscle fiber in cardiovascular exercise?"

Easy. Give your muscles more resistance. Perform smarter interval training. That's how exercising less leads to fat loss and cardiovascular health.

Brian Irving, PhD, of the University of Virginia, took two groups of women and had them do traditional cardiovascular exercise or smarter cardiovascular exercise. The two groups burned the same number of calories exercising, but the smarter-exercise group spent significantly less time exercising, while losing significantly more belly fat.[170]

Martin Gibala, PhD, of McMaster University, separated people into smarter cardiovascular exercise and traditional cardiovascular exercise groups. Over the course of the two-week study, the Smarter Group exercised for two-and-a-half hours while the traditional exercise group exercised for ten-and-a-half hours. At the end of the study both groups got the same results even though the smarter-exercise group spent 320 percent less time exercising than the traditional exercise group. Gibala put it like this: "We thought there would be benefits, but we did not expect them to be this obvious. It shows how effective short intense exercise can be." [171]

Many more studies show the same encouraging results and further prove that hours spent exercising per week are unnecessary when compared with smarter exercise. Consider this small sample:

- A study at Harvard University found that "vigorous activities are associated with a reduced risk of coronary heart disease, whereas moderate or light activities have no clear association with the risk of coronary heart disease." [172]
- A study at Stanford University found that "the intensity of effort was more important than the quantity of energy output in deterring hypertension and preventing premature mortality." [173]
- Another study from Harvard found that "there is an inverse association between relative intensity of physical activity and risk of coronary heart disease." [174]
- The American Heart Association noted that "vigorous-intensity activities may have greater benefit for reducing cardiovascular disease and premature mortality than moderate-intensity physical activities." [175]
- Researchers at the Norwegian University of Science and Technology discovered that "exercise training reduces the impact of the metabolic syndrome [the clog] and that the magnitude of the effect depends on exercise intensity [quality]." [176]

Even day-to-day cardiovascular benefits, like not being out of breath after walking up a few flights of stairs, are achieved faster with smarter exercise. Edward Coyle, PhD, in the Department of Kinesiology and Health Education at the University of Texas, found that interval training produced a marked increase in aerobic endurance among untrained people, serving as "a dramatic reminder of the potency of exercise intensity."[177] Vigorous intensity exercise has been shown to increase aerobic fitness more effectively than moderate intensity exercise, and this fact hints at its greater cardio-protective effects as well. If you like doing cardio, then smarter interval training has clearly emerged as the best way to spend your time. You can trade quantity for quality and get more for less by increasing the force of your exercise. (Again, we will cover exactly how to do this in part 3.)

PRINCIPLE 6: HEAL—DON'T HURT—YOURSELF

Given how little time eccentric and smarter interval training takes, a common reaction to this new approach to exercise is: "Sounds good. I'll just add that to my existing routine." That might not necessarily be a bad approach, but to ensure that we spend our time healing rather than harming ourselves, it is critical to keep four things in mind:

1. Unless it is a very-low-intensity and low-impact activity such as walking or yoga, more isn't better; it's worse.
2. Spare time is best spent on sleep, increasing the SANEity of your eating program, and then on restorative and recreational activities.
3. The safest and most sustainable way to increase intensity is to increase resistance while *decreasing* speed.
4. Protect your time, money, and mind.

MORE ISN'T BETTER; IT'S WORSE

Imagine you recently had major surgery and have been prescribed a cutting-edge prescription to help you heal. Your surgeon tells you to take one dose per week. At one dose per week this prescription will make you quite sore, but will benefit you in ways that are hard to believe until you experience them. She then informs you that because of its high potency it is critical not to increase the dose. You get it. You keep your recovery simple. You stay patient while your body heals itself. And you enjoy a healthier and happier version of yourself for the rest of your life.

Smarter exercise is similar. Owing to its high potency, more is not better; it's worse. There are few areas in life where we have the opportunity to do less and get more. Pharmacology and physiology are two of them. Take advantage of this opportunity. You have access to the world's most powerful physiological prescription for hormonal healing. Take it as prescribed. Keep your recovery simple. Stay patient. Let your body heal itself. And then enjoy a healthier and happier version of yourself for the rest of your life.

SPARE TIME IS BEST SPENT ON SLEEP AND ENJOYABLE ACTIVITIES

If you want to use the spare time freed up thanks to exercising less—but smarter—on your health, you would be best served spending it (in order of benefit):

1. Sleeping more. I know this seems like common sense, but consider one of the most frequently prescribed methods to burn fat and boost health: sleep less, exercise more. Hormonally clogged, sleep-deprived, and overstressed individuals are told to wake up early to further stress their body. This worsens their hormonal clog. Telling us to wake up at 4:00 a.m. and jog for an hour is like telling someone who just broke an ankle to stop icing it and to go jump up and down on it.

   Remember, a broken metabolism really is like a broken ankle: *it heals itself* when we put less stress on it—not more. Sleeping less increases stress. Traditional exercise increases stress. Starvation increases stress. That's why we're going to eat more and exercise less—but smarter—and take the time we save and spend it sleeping. We're going to figuratively rest, ice, elevate, and do a little physical therapy to enable our broken metabolism to heal itself.

2. Increasing the quality of your eating. Think of creative ways to maximize your intake of exceptionally SANE foods such as deep leafy greens, seafood, grass-fed meats, cocoa/cacao, coconut, acai berries, goji berries, green tea, etc. Remember, the quality of the food we eat is at least 90 percent of the long-term health and fitness equation.

3. Enjoying very low-intensity and low-impact restorative and relaxing activities such as walking, recreational bike riding, yoga, Pilates, stretching, tai chi, meditation, qigong, etc. Moving more is wonderful for you as long as it reduces stress. Do about a half hour of eccentric and smarter interval training per week and then focus on restorative activities.

4. Doing exercise-related hobbies such as jogging or going to an aerobics class with friends in moderation. If a moderate amount of traditional exercise helps you reduce stress and makes you happy, then by all means enjoy it. However, please do not let it have a negative impact on your smarter exercise, SANEity, sleep, or emotional state.

Here's what not to do. Sleep less so that you can jog for two hours on hard pavement while breathing in car exhaust. Quench your thirst with a "sports drink" whose primary ingredient is high-fructose corn syrup. Eat a plate of pasta and breadsticks because of your postjog starchy-carb cravings. Treat yourself to some ice cream, since you "deserve it" for jogging. Sleep even less the next night because of the insomnia those inSANE foods caused. Wake up the next day feeling terrible, skip your eccentrics because you are sore, binge on inSANE sweets because you are overstressed, and then max out your credit card buying pills, powders, and potions that promise to make everything better because you feel that despite trying harder, you are doing worse. You are not broken. The "eat less, then sleep less so you can exercise more" approach is broken. Go smarter, not harder, and you will transform your life more simply and affordably than you ever thought possible.

INCREASE RESISTANCE WHILE DECREASING SPEED

Every few years, a new at-home "extreme" workout video will come out. These workouts attempt to increase intensity by increasing the speed of exercise. We jump, we sprint, we flail around, and we work up a sweat, but we do not work all our muscle fibers, and we do set ourselves up to get seriously injured.

When you exercise smarter, you will be completely exhausted in a matter of seconds. That's intense. You will do that by moving in an extremely slow and controlled manner. That's safe. You will put zero impact on your joints. That's sustainable. You will be sore for several days after a single short workout. That's effective. Smarter exercise actually does what these videos claim to do and it does so dramatically more safely and sustainably.

It may be helpful to think of these videos and other extreme forms of exercise as a bit like cutting your hair with a chainsaw. It may sort of work, but it also carries along with it excessive and unnecessary risk. Also, if these exercises were as potent as they claim, why would we need to do them five to seven days per week? Think about the potency of exercise as being like the potency of an ingredient in a recipe. We do not need a large quantity of potent things—and if we need a lot of something, it is not potent. Eccentric exercise, done for a few minutes once per week, actually is potent exercise.

To be fair, quite a few young athletic people swear by these extreme-exercise regimens. If you enjoy extreme exercise and can do it safely without craving starches and sweets or skimping on your eccentrics, then by all means, enjoy. Let's just make sure we're doing what's best for our health and fitness for the rest of our lives.

When it comes to evaluating the long-term efficacy of exercise, there are three primary criteria to look at (in priority order):

1. Safety
2. Sustainability
3. Resistance

SAFETY: If an exercise technique isn't safe, it's counterproductive. Let's say Tom slips a disk in his back while powerlifting and can't resistance-train effectively for the rest of his life. Some people like to say, "Pain is temporary, pride is forever." As someone who was part of a state championship Ohio football team and also blew his knee out twice playing football, I can tell you that pride is temporary, pain is forever. Talking about my high school successes grew old many years ago, but my knee still hurts.

SUSTAINABILITY: If an exercise technique isn't sustainable, it risks being counterproductive. Back in my football days, we did workouts at 6:00 a.m. and then again in the afternoon. Both of these workouts made mainstream extreme workouts look relaxing. Vomiting and passing out were quite common. Today, just about every one of my teammates and I no longer train even close to that way either because we got hurt doing it or because it was so absurd that it spoiled exercise for us. This is one of the reasons why some former athletes become obese. Unsustainable approaches can lead to burnout and complete exercise avoidance long term.

RESISTANCE: Increasing exercise resistance (versus duration or frequency) is the key to hormonal healing. If an exercise technique doesn't allow us to easily add resistance, the only way to increase intensity is to do the movement faster and that is a recipe for injury. This is why running isn't as good as stationary biking when it comes to smarter exercise—it's quite difficult to safely add a lot of resistance while running.

Before you try any new exercise program, I recommend asking yourself three questions:

1. Does this put safety first?
2. Can I do this for the rest of my life?
3. Can I increase resistance without increasing risk?

If you answer no to any of these questions, you may want to stick with eccentrics and smarter intervals.

If you take nothing else from this book, please remember this statement:

There is no pill, product, or service that comes close to providing the health and physique benefits you will get from eating so many non-starchy vegetables, nutrient-dense proteins, and whole-food fats that you are too full for starches and sweets.

Why do I say this? At least 95 percent of people avoided obesity and over 99 percent avoided diabetes for all human history before (insert name of new pill, product, or service) existed. Remember, slim is simple, but there is a massive amount of money to be made in convincing us otherwise.

Until we achieve baseline health and fitness, anything or anyone who makes avoiding obesity and disease seem more complex than eating more but higher-quality food, and doing less but higher-quality exercise, should be ignored. Otherwise, we will end up heavier, sicker, and with less money in the long term.

Of course if we are already healthy and fit and now want to achieve unnaturally low levels of body fat or world-class athletic performance, we should absolutely get our credit cards out and get ready for some complexity. But if our goal is to be slim and healthy for the rest of our lives, the most effective way to do that is to keep things simple, SANE, eccentric, and inexpensive.

We've learned the science of the set-point. We've seen how we can eat more—but smarter—by going SANE. And we've discovered how we can exercise less—but smarter—by getting eccentric and by doing smarter intervals. Now that we know how we make our body transform itself by eating and exercising smarter, it's time to make our mind transform itself by thinking smarter.

Just as putting high-quality food into our body dramatically enhances our ability to reach our goals, putting high-quality thoughts into our mind dramatically enhances our ability to reach our goals, too. Part 3 covers a specific five-week plan that will create a beautiful mind along with a beautiful body and empower you along a lifetime of previously unimaginable vitality.

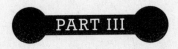

PART III

THE
SANE SOLUTION
AND
ACTION PLAN

Thought is the sculptor who can create the person you want to be.

—Henry David Thoreau

23

Smarter Subconscious

Everything is easier when our subconscious is on our side. A 24/7/365 internal monologue affirming that we will reach and maintain our wellness goals is critical to success. As the saying goes: "Sow a thought and you reap an action; sow an act and you reap a habit; sow a habit and you reap a character; sow a character and you reap a destiny."

The first step we can take to develop a smarter subconscious is to think in terms of utilitarianism. Utilitarians are focused on pleasure and pain. They believe something is good to the extent it provides the most pleasure and avoids the most pain for the most people. They also make a distinction between the various types of pleasure. Compare the pleasure of watching a loved one accomplish a long-sought-after goal versus the pleasure of taking a nap. Utilitarianism and common sense tell us some pleasures bring deeper and longer-term joy than others. While pleasures of the senses—tastes, touches, smells, sounds, and sights—are nice, they are not as good as pleasures of the mind or spirit: spending time with friends and family, solving a complex problem, reaching a goal, and similar soul-nourishing endeavors.

This framework is a helpful starting point to shift our subconscious as it shows how SANEity provides us with the most pleasure and avoids the most pain. Consider these two versions of Sally.

SANE Sally eats more and exercises less—but smarter—while treating herself to sweets and starches once a week. Sally feels and looks great. This gives her a deep and long-term sense of satisfaction and accomplishment. This radiates in every aspect of her life. Her demeanor, energy level, mental sharpness, and body confidence not only make her feel great but also are obvious and impressive to those around her.

InSANE Sally eats mostly starches and sweets and is inactive. While eating this way does bring her some brief pleasure, she feels terrible for most of the day and she doesn't feel good about herself. She is borderline depressed, constantly feels sick, suffers from mysterious aches and pains, has little energy, can't think clearly, and isn't as pleasant with her family, friends, and coworkers as she could be. This causes her, and those around her, significant distress.

From the utilitarian standpoint, being SANE and smart is the most pleasurable option available to us. We trade shallow short-term pleasure that causes deep long-term pain for more meaningful long-term pleasure.

Next, we can leverage the technique popularized by Dr. Nathaniel Branden known as sentence completion. All we do is write an incomplete sentence and then add a series of different endings. In his book *The Six Pillars of Self-Esteem*, Branden writes, "Sentence-completion work is a deceptively simple yet uniquely powerful tool for raising self-understanding, self-esteem, and personal effectiveness. It rests on the premise that all of us have more knowledge than we normally are aware of—more wisdom than we use, more potential than typically shows up in our behavior. Sentence completion is a tool for accessing and activating these 'hidden resources.'"[178]

For example, consider the following incomplete sentences:

When I slim down and tone up, I am excited to: _____ .

When I slim down and tone up, I will feel: _____ .

When I have more energy, my relationship with _____ will improve because: _____ .

When I have more energy, _____'s life will improve because: _____ .

Here are the same sentences, each completed a few times.

When I slim down and tone up, I am excited to *buy sassy new clothes*.

When I slim down and tone up, I am excited to *see the expression on my friends' faces*.

When I slim down and tone up, I will feel *more confident*.

When I slim down and tone up, I will feel *proud of myself*.

When I have more energy, my relationship with my *partner* will improve because *I won't be crabby when I get home from work*.

When I have more energy, my relationship with *my friends* will improve because *I'll be able to spend more time with them, since I'll get my work done quicker*.

When I have more energy, *my kids'* lives will improve because *I'll be able to play with them outside*.

When I have more energy, *my* life will improve because *I'll perform better at my job and get that raise I deserve*.

Consistently completing sentences like this is powerful because it changes what our subconscious perceives as pleasurable and painful.

Seem like a stretch? Have you ever noticed how it's not only easy but enjoyable for vegans to avoid all animal products? Most people would find forgoing all animal products terribly painful, but most vegans find it pleasurable. How do they do this?

When someone sets a steak in front of them, their mind quickly makes a pro/con list that is heavily stacked in favor of sticking to their principles. See the illustration on page 200.

Vegans effortlessly skip the succulent steak because doing so is the most pleasurable option.

What if we could make our minds work in the same, effortless way, but for inSANE food instead? What if we got more pleasure from avoiding inSANE food than we got from eating it? Then it would feel much better to savor a SANE peanut butter mousse dessert (see Recipes, page 240) than eat a box of doughnuts. So how can we get our minds to work this way?

Sentence completion is one useful tool. It helps us develop a subconscious packed full of reasons that "meaningful long-term pleasure comes from SANE foods" while "meaningful long-term pain comes from inSANE starches and sweets." As the weeks of SANE eating and smarter exercise roll by and your body, mood, health, and energy levels dra-

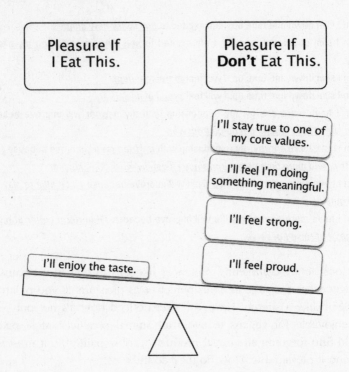

matically improve, your results will speak for themselves, and will serve as positive reinforcement, making it easy to stay on track.

Smarter Sentence Completion, Part 1

Think of sentence completion as a simple do-it-yourself version of the visualization exercises elite athletes are coached through. By deliberately rehearsing something in our mind, we can restructure our brain without having to physically accomplish the action. This neurological restructuring not only gives us the confidence and motivation to reach our goals but also helps us to develop sustainable habits much more quickly. Long term, I recommend sprinkling in a few minutes of sentence completion once per week. To get started, spend no more than fifteen minutes completing the following sentences ten times each. The only requirements are that you spend a maximum of fifteen seconds on each sentence, avoid censoring yourself, and complete the exercise in one undisturbed sitting at the very start or end of your day. Think of it as a written meditation. Let your thoughts flow freely. Enjoy the exercise.

When I slim down and tone up, I am excited to: _____ .
When I slim down and tone up, I will be: _____ .
When I slim down and tone up, _____ 's life will improve because:
_____
When I slim down and tone up, I will feel: _____ .
When I slim down and tone up, my relationship with _____
will improve because: _____ .

Short term, work through the sentence-completion exercises in the next two sections in half-hour chunks. I think that you'll find these exercises to be a powerful tool for creating a lifestyle that is happier and healthier.

Smarter Sentence Completion, Part 2

If you just finished some sentence-completion exercises, skip ahead to the next chapter. Do the sentence-completion exercises in this section and the next section over the next two days. It's best if you don't spend more than a half hour per day on sentence completion. Remember to complete each of the following sentences ten times quickly. We want to rely on our subconscious, not our conscious mind. Spend a maximum of fifteen seconds on each sentence.

When I have more energy, I am excited to: _____ .
When I have more energy, I will be: _____ .
When I have more energy, _____ 's life will improve because:
_____
When I have more energy, I will feel: _____ .
When I have more energy, my relationship with _____
will improve because: _____ .
When I am tempted to eat inSANEly, I will remember_____
and pick a more SANE option.
Avoiding major degenerative diseases such as cancer, heart disease, diabetes, etc.,
would be nice because: _____ .
By setting a smarter example, I: _____ .

Smarter Sentence Completion, Part 3

When I feel better about myself, I am excited to: _____ .

When I feel better about myself, I will be: _____ .

When I feel better about myself, _____ 's life will improve because:

_____ .

When I feel better about myself, my relationship with _____

will improve because: _____ .

Living twenty years longer would be nice because: _____ .

Having ten extra hours per week thanks to exercising smarter would improve

_____

because: _____ .

When I have fewer aches and pains, I am excited to: _____ .

When I have fewer aches and pains, my relationship with _____

will improve because: _____ .

Ongoing Smarter Sentence Completion

At the end of each of your five weeks to SANEity (see the next chapter), set aside twenty minutes to do a fresh batch of these sentence-completion exercises.

This week I am proud that I: _____ .

This week I noticed that eating more and exercising less—smarter—had a positive impact on my life when: _____ .

This week I noticed that eating more and exercising less—smarter—had a positive impact on _____ 's life when:

_____ .

Next week I will be excited to eat more and exercise less—smarter—because:

_____ .

24

Five Weeks to Complete SANEity

Earlier we applied the teachings of the eighteenth-century German philosopher Immanuel Kant to fat loss and health. We covered how anything we do to boost wellness must be continued or our health will suffer. Therefore, we should skip any wellness program that we cannot keep up forever. A seven-day cleanse may be challenging, but what happens on day eight?

With Kant's philosophy in mind, we're going to ease our way into our new lifestyle. "Calm, gradual, and patient" is the right formula for the long term; all-or-nothing approaches are doomed to failure. Compare trying to be more active by attempting to run ten miles right now versus walking five more minutes every day while slowly adding pep to your step. Which is more likely to help you be more active in the long term? Remember, we're focused on the next thirty years and beyond, not the next thirty days.

With a lifetime of fitness in mind, we're going to make simple changes to the way we eat and exercise over five weeks. Each week we will swap a few more starches and sweets for a few more nonstarchy vegetables, nutrient-dense proteins, whole-food fats, and low-fructose fruits, and we'll add a little more resistance to our smarter exercise. We'll use a simple food tracker to keep general tabs on what we're eating (see the table on page 204). The black squares represent a serv-

FIVE WEEKS TO COMPLETE SANEity AND A LOWER SET-POINT

(Gray = Optional, Black = Required)

			Week 1	Week 2
SANE	Nonstarchy Vegetables	Ate:	□□□□□□□□□□□□□	□□□□□□□□□□□□□
		Target:	■■■■■▨▨▨▨▨▨▨▨	■■■■■▨▨▨▨▨▨▨▨
	Nutrient-Dense Protein	Ate:	□□□□□□□□□□□□□	□□□□□□□□□□□□□
		Target:	■■■■▨▨	■■■■■▨
	Whole-Food Fats	Ate:	□□□□□□□□□□□□□	□□□□□□□□□□□□□
		Target:	■■▨▨	■■■▨
	Low-Fructose Fruits	Ate:	□□□□□□□□□□□□□	□□□□□□□□□□□□□
		Target:	▨▨▨▨▨▨	▨▨▨▨▨
	Legumes	Ate:	□□□□□□□□□□□□□	□□□□□□□□□□□□□
		Target:	▨▨▨	▨▨▨
	Other Fruits	Ate:	□□□□□□□□□□□□□	□□□□□□□□□□□□□
		Target:	▨▨▨▨	▨▨▨
	Most Dairy	Ate:	□□□□□□□□□□□□□	□□□□□□□□□□□□□
		Target:	▨▨▨▨	▨▨▨
	Other Fats	Ate:	□□□□□□□□□□□□□	□□□□□□□□□□□□□
		Target:	▨▨▨▨	▨▨▨
inSANE	Starch	Ate:	□□□□□□□□□□□□□	□□□□□□□□□□□□□
		Target:	▨▨▨▨▨▨	▨▨▨▨▨
	Sweet/ Sweetened Drinks	Ate:	□□□□□□□□□□□□□	□□□□□□□□□□□□□
		Target:	▨▨▨	▨▨▨

ing of a food we need to lower our set-point. Gray squares represent a serving of a food we can eat if we would like to. The empty squares are what we check off when we eat.

It may be helpful to make copies of the food tracker so you can check off the boxes day by day. Be sure to also get your free companion app at www.SANESolution.com to help track and optimize your SANEity. Additionally, keep in mind that it is OK to eat more nonstarchy vegetables. The tracker shows daily minimums for nonstarchy vegetables. The more nonstarchy vegetables we eat, the healthier and slimmer we will be.

Also keep in mind that just as we want to avoid hunger, we also want to avoid feeling uncomfortably full. Use this tracker as a guide, but listen to your body. If you are not hungry and are on track to eat

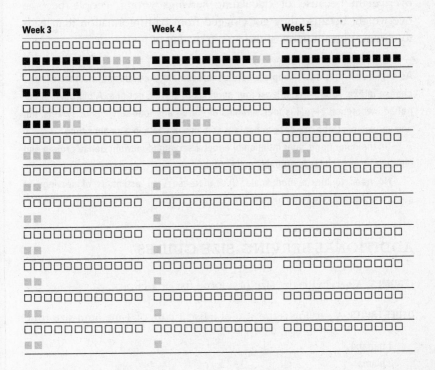

at least three 30-gram servings of protein and at least eight servings of nonstarchy vegetables and some essential fats, you do not need to make yourself uncomfortably full. Use the serving-size guidelines we outlined earlier for nonstarchy vegetables, nutrient-dense protein, whole-food fats, and low-fructose fruits. In a few pages we'll look at some additional guidelines to help determine how many serving boxes you should check each time you eat. Also, note that the serving-size information given on food labels is generally accurate. To see this for yourself, look at a container of your favorite starch or sweet and note how tiny a serving size is.

Keep in mind that everything related to serving sizes and number of servings that we cover here is a general guideline. It is easy to get mired in details and to complicate things in talking about servings and serving sizes. Let's stay focused on the big picture and use these guidelines to estimate our intake as accurately as we can. Nobody is overweight because of calculating servings wrong. People become overweight because they got clogged from bad information that leads to chronic consumption of the wrong quality of food.

As a general rule, most people wildly underestimate their starch, sweets, oil, and cheese intake. A bagel is at least four servings of starch, not one. A big bowl of enriched sweetened cereal is four servings of starch and four servings of sweets, not one serving of starch. It's easy to eat four servings of pasta in a single sitting.

On the other hand, your intuition of about a serving of nutrient-dense protein and nonstarchy vegetables is probably quite close.

No need to buy a food scale. Just increase your estimates of servings of starches, sweets, oils, and cheeses.

ADDITIONAL SERVING-SIZE GUIDES

LEGUMES: A serving is the size of a loose fist or 1 cup.

OTHER FRUITS: A serving is the size of a fist, 1 cup, or 1 medium-size fruit.

1 banana
2 plums
15 grapes
1 apple
1 peach

MOST DAIRY: A serving of butter is the size of the tip of your thumb (one teaspoon). A serving of cheese is about the size of your thumb. A serving of milk or high-sugar yogurt is 1 cup (eight ounces). Most people could easily eat four servings of butter or cheese but only a serving or two of milk or yogurt in a sitting. Baked goods can saturate you with butter before you know it. Every time you eat pizza, you are likely to be eating over four servings of cheese. Butter and cheese are easy to overeat.

OTHER FATS: An extremely fatty cut of conventional meat the size of your palm is two or three servings. One teaspoon of oil is also a serving.

Aside from a few guys trying to prove something, most people would stop eating fatty meat naturally at two or three servings in a single sitting. However, it is extremely easy to overeat oil. Eat anything fried and you will easily consume at least four servings of oil.

STARCHY VEGETABLES/STARCH: Serving sizes vary. The key point is that a serving of starch is small. For example, a bag of popcorn can easily contain eight servings. Starches are extremely easy to overeat because they are dry and low in fiber and protein. Most people overeat starch daily without knowing it. When ranchers want to fatten livestock, they stop feeding them nonstarchy plants (grass) and start feeding them starch (generally corn). If you do not want to fatten yourself, avoid starch, especially in these common excess quantities.

bagel ⟶ at least 4 servings
muffins ⟶ at least 3 servings
baked potato ⟶ at least 3 servings
french fries ⟶ at least 4 servings
a traditional portion of pasta or rice ⟶ at least 4 servings
a traditional bowl of cereal ⟶ at least 4 servings
baked goods ⟶ at least 4 servings

SWEETS/SWEETENED DRINKS: Ten grams of "sugar" (anything *with calories* that is *added* to food to make it sweeter) is a serving. Sweets are the easiest food to overeat. Some sweeteners aren't even recognized as food by the body and never trigger a full feeling. This is why you can take in three servings of sweets by drinking a soda and still have plenty of room for a pink slime burger and fries cooked in toxic trans fats. Traditional portions of sweets and sweetened drinks contain three to eight servings. The fastest way to gain fat and damage your health is to eat and drink sweeteners.

can of soda ⟶ at least 3 servings
desserts ⟶ at least 4 servings
a traditional bowl of sweetened cereal ⟶ at least 4 servings
fruit juice ⟶ at least 3 servings

A SAMPLE DAY

Before we move on to the smarter exercise program, let's look at a typical day on a SANE eating program, with typical foods and serving estimations for what you'll be eating. Again, note that the serving sizes are intentionally approximations. Please don't sweat the small stuff. As Dr. John Yudkin, of the University of London, puts it, "There is no point in worrying about imaginary dangers. If you do, you will be likely to go on overlooking the real dangers." [179] Dedicate all your attention to healing your body with at least ten servings of nonstarchy vegetables, 100 to 200 grams of protein in at least 30-gram doses, whole-food fats, low-fructose fruits, and smarter exercise. Your body is miraculous—it will take care of the rest.

What I Ate Today:	SMART Translation:
Breakfast: 2 eggs and 6 egg whites scrambled with a lot of vegetables and ham, green tea	1.5 nutrient-dense protein, 3 nonstarchy vegetables, 1 whole-food fat
Lunch: Stir-fried chicken with a lot of vegetables, green tea	1.5 nutrient-dense protein, 1 other fat, 3 nonstarchy vegetables
Optional snacks: SANE pancakes, raw-sugar snap peas and baby carrots, green smoothie, drinking lots of water	1 whole-food fat, 1 nutrient-dense protein, 4 nonstarchy vegetables
Dinner: A lot of baked salmon, grilled vegetables, decaf green tea, SANE peanut butter mousse	2 nutrient-dense protein, 3 nonstarchy vegetables, 3 whole-food fats

TOTAL NUTRITION FOR THE DAY

	Servings
Nonstarchy Vegetables	13
Nutrient-Dense Protein	6
Whole-Food Fats	6
Low-Fructose Fruits	1
Legumes	
Other Fruits	
Most Dairy	

Other	
Fats	1
Starch	
Sweets/Sweetened Drinks	

We will cover a full week of SANE recipes and how to simplify cooking shortly, but first let's explore our smarter exercise program.

Is SANE Eating the Same for Children and Adults?

Yes and no. Yes, in that the same foods are SANE for children and adults. No, in that eating Satisfying, unAggressive, Nutritious, and inEfficient food is *more* important for children because

- Children require more nutrition than adults.
- Children are more susceptible to food-related behavior problems.
- Fat cells never go away.
- The habits children form affect them forever.

Children Require More Nutrition Than Adults

Water-, fiber-, and protein-rich foods contain more nutrition per calorie than any other foods. A SANE child is optimizing growth and development with the most essential vitamins, minerals, proteins, and fats possible.

Some children may also require an abundance of calories. The research clearly shows that we're best off supplying extra calories via whole-food fats rather than starches or sweets (this applies to athletes as well). This can be done deliciously by enjoying more of the SANE desserts we'll cover shortly, or simply by adding cocoa/cacao, coconut, avocado, flax seeds, or chia seeds to smoothies.

Children Are More Susceptible to Food-Related Behavior Problems

Starches and sweets are dramatically more Aggressive than SANE foods. They release a short burst of energy into the body. This causes a brief energy high followed by longer-lasting lethargy. Still developing mentally and emotionally, children are doubly affected by these highs and lows; that is why they start bouncing off the walls and have a hard time concentrating after eating starches and sweets.

SANEr eating has long been "prescribed" to aid children said to be suffering from ADHD (attention deficit hyperactivity disorder), as it ensures a slow and steady supply of energy and enables optimal mood and behavior.

Fat Cells Never Go Away

Once fat cells are made, we cannot get rid of them; we can only shrink them. This is why helping our children avoid excess body fat is so important and why childhood obesity is so heartbreaking. Once a child develops new fat cells, he will have a harder time staying slim *for the rest of his life* because those fat cells will never go away. They can be shrunk, but will forever predispose that child to storing excess body fat. In fact, the American Heart Association found that 70 to 80 percent of overweight children remain overweight their entire lives.[180]

The Habits Children Form Affect Them Forever

The habits we learn as children stick with us. When we teach our children healthy habits, we make it dramatically easier for them to keep themselves fit and healthy for the rest of their lives.

Simple SANE Cooking

At the end of this chapter we'll review a full week of recipes that includes options for breakfast, lunch, dinner, snacks, and dessert, but before we go there let's keep SANE cooking simple by cooking in bulk and savoring substitutions for starches and sweets.

COOK IN BULK

Just as buying nonstarchy vegetables, nutrient-dense protein, whole-food fats, and low-fructose fruits in bulk will save you thousands of dollars over the course of a year, cooking in bulk will save you hundreds of hours over the course of a year. I like to talk about cooking in the same way that we talked about tea. Much as there is $4 per bag tea and $0.04 per bag tea, we can spend three hours cooking a single meal or we can spend twenty minutes cooking a delicious SANE dish that we can enjoy five times. We are going to focus on the latter. If you enjoy the former, keep it up, and stay SANE by making the starch and sweet substitutions we'll cover in a moment.

Given our goal of preparing scrumptious SANE food as time- and cost-efficiently as possible, we're going to need some big bowls and some storage containers because we're going to be making big batches and freezing a lot of it. At the very least, every time you cook, prepare two meals: one you will eat now and one you will eat later. Many people take this two steps further and create four meals every time they cook: one that they enjoy immediately, another that they enjoy the next day, and two meals' worth that they freeze and enjoy the following week. By following this routine we can significantly reduce the amount of time we spend in the kitchen.

SAVORY SUBSTITUTIONS FOR STARCHES AND SWEETS

Staying SANE isn't about deprivation. It's about enjoying so much good food that we're too full for the sickening stuff. Even better, there are a lot of delicious foods that aren't starches or sweets. In fact, studies show that chocolate is the most craved food in the world,' and the ingredient that puts the "c" in chocolate—cocoa/cacao—is spectacularly SANE.

Keeping the "substitution rather than deprivation" principle in mind, we can cook and eat almost anything by making some simple swaps. While these swaps will taste slightly different, they will also make us look and feel completely different—a trade-off that you will very much enjoy long term. The cheat sheet below will get you started SANEly swapping your way to slimness.

I refer to a specific product called UMP made by Beverly International in some of the charts and recipes in this chapter. I am in no way being compensated by this company for this recommendation. I mention this specific product because I have not found another protein powder that cooks as well as this product does. I highly recommend sticking with this specific product if you choose to enjoy the recipes that refer to it. Think of it as SANE flour, cake batter, pancake batter, etc.

SANE SWAP CHEAT SHEET

inSANE	SANE
pasta and rice	• spaghetti squash/Squoodles
	• zucchini noodles/Zoodles
	• shirataki noodles
	• shredded cabbage
	• shaved brussels sprouts
	• bean sprouts
	• pea shoots
	• cauliflower rice
	• broccoli and carrot slaw (premade in grocery produce section)

potatoes	• mashed cauliflower
	• turnips
	• eggplant
	• squash
	• zucchini
bread, cookies, cakes, pies, waffles, pancakes, and tortillas	• baked goods made using golden flaxseed meal, coconut flour, almond meal, almond flour, and other nut flours
	• low-carb and diabetic breads, tortillas, etc., that contain as few ingredients as possible, UMP
hot and cold cereal	• SANE cereals made with ground flax, nuts, and chia. (See recipes in the next section.)
pretzels and chips	• nuts
	• seeds
	• baked kale chips

ONE WEEK OF SANE EATING

Remember the former top English pastry chef turned SANE chef we met earlier? Here is a full week of SANE recipes and snacks from Carrie Brown herself.

For many of the recipes that follow you will find SANE and SANEst versions. If eating foods that taste as good as possible is your primary goal and burning fat and boosting health are secondary, stick with the SANE options. If burning fat and boosting your health as quickly as possible are your primary goal and enjoying delicious food is secondary, go with the SANEst option. Or mix it up. Or customize the recipes to best fit your goals. Do what works best for you.

The SANE desserts are optional but delicious. The SANEst versions of them are so healthy that they can also be used as snacks or meals as long as we make sure we get our nonstarchy vegetables elsewhere. The snacks are also optional. The only thing to keep in mind is the 30-grams-of-protein thresholds (if you are living a low-carb SANE lifestyle, it is fine to use full-fat low-sugar dairy and whole eggs). It's more metabolically beneficial to enjoy 30 grams of protein in a single sitting than 15 grams in two separate sittings.

You will find both simple and more elaborate recipes here to reflect the diversity of options available to us. If you like to keep things simple, you can use this general formula: choose lots of nonstarchy vegetables and seafood or nutrient-dense meat, and some whole-food fats and/or low-fructose fruits as dessert. For example, lots of grilled asparagus and eggplant along with a grass-fed steak or salmon followed up with SANE chocolate peanut butter fudge. Drink at least sixteen ounces of water or green tea with the meal.

Do your best to eat only when you are truly hungry. You can test this by drinking twelve ounces of water or green tea, waiting five minutes, and seeing if you are still hungry. Your body will be fueling itself with your stored body fat so you will be surprised at how little hunger you feel between meals. If you cannot comfortably eat the number of servings of SANE nonstarchy vegetables, nutrient-dense protein, and whole-food fats outlined earlier, it is OK to eat less only if you never get hungry and if you are not "saving room" for starches and sweets. If at the end of a day you have eaten eight servings of nonstarchy vegetables, three 30-gram servings of nutrient-dense protein, and three servings of natural fats and are completely full and satisfied, that's fine. However, if this causes you to crave starches and sweets in between meals and after 9 p.m., then eat more SANE food.

When you do eat, enjoy yourself. Eat until you are completely satisfied and then stop. A simple way to do this is to eat slowly and to pause and relax for five minutes when you start to feel satisfied. You should never feel hungry or uncomfortably full while living SANEly.

Here's a sample menu for one week of eating SANEly:

MONDAY
Breakfast
> Strawberry–Chia Seed Cereal
> Strawberry-Avocado Green Smoothie

Lunch
> Broccoli and Red Pepper Miniquiches
> Cinnamon and Raisin "Rice" Pudding

Dinner

Turkey and Mushroom Stroganoff

Squash Noodles

Dessert

Peanut Butter Mousse

TUESDAY

Breakfast

Grain-Free Granola

Super Yogurt

Orange Creamsicle Green Smoothie

Lunch

Large dark green salad with two hard-boiled eggs

Dinner

Turkey and Almond Stir-Fry

Dessert

Mint Chocolate Pudding

WEDNESDAY

Breakfast

Vanilla Almond Hot Cereal

Strawberry-Avocado Green Smoothie

Lunch

Leek and Cauliflower Soup

Cottage cheese mixed with diced ham or turkey

Dinner

Prawn and Mushroom Stir-Fry

Dessert

Chocolate-Covered Berry Cream

THURSDAY

Breakfast

German Chocolate Pancakes

Orange Creamsicle Green Smoothie

Lunch

Peanut Butter–Chicken Salad, served over spinach

Dinner

Lasagna

Dessert

Chocolate–Peanut Butter Fudge

FRIDAY

Breakfast

Almond Pear Cereal

Strawberry-Avocado Green Smoothie

Lunch

Large dark green salad with salmon burgers

Creamy Cucumber Soup

Dinner

Chicken Carbonara

Dessert

Caramel-Orange-Spice Cashews

SATURDAY

Breakfast

Ham and Eggs Bake

Spinach or kale, onions, mushrooms, and peppers stir-fried in coconut oil

Lunch

Smoked Salmon and Bean Sprout Sauté

Dinner

Pork Chops with Bacon and Cabbage

Zucchini and Cherry Tomato Salad

Dessert

Orange-Cranberry Scones

SUNDAY

Breakfast

Omelet filled with as much of your favorite nonstarchy vegetables as possible

Lunch

Chicken, Avocado, and Walnut Salad

Dinner

Salmon with Orange and Fennel

Mixed green salad

Almond Parmesan Squash

Dessert

Dark Chocolate–Espresso Cookies

SANE SNACKS

If you are hungry, you may snack whenever you wish. Here are some examples of SANE snack choices:

- handful of raw nuts + unprocessed lunch meat and/or raw nonstarchy vegetables
- 30 g of protein worth of hard boiled eggs and egg whites (example: 5 whole eggs, 8 egg whites, 2 whole eggs and 5 egg whites, etc.)
- 1 to 3 cups raw nonstarchy vegetables such as sugar snap peas, celery, carrots, cucumber, broccoli with plain Greek yogurt dip
- 30 g of protein worth of unprocessed lunch meat
- 30 g of protein worth of beef, turkey, or salmon jerky
- 30 g of protein worth of cottage cheese (a heaping cup full) mixed with ¾ cup berries

- 30 g of protein worth of plain Greek yogurt (a heaping cup) mixed with ¾ cup berries
- protein bar with at least 30 g protein and less than 8 g sugar (example: one and a half Quest bars)
- 30 g of protein worth of SANE pancakes, German chocolate pancakes, "rice" pudding, peanut butter mousse, or super yogurt
- 30 g of protein worth of sardines (example: approximately two packages depending on the brand)
- Green smoothie

THE RECIPES
Breakfast

Almond Pear Cereal

Makes 2 servings

SANE	SANEst
2 large, firm pears, cored and roughly chopped	No Change
⅔ cup light coconut milk	No Change
1 cup almond meal	No Change
¼ cup ground flaxseed	No Change
⅔ cup vanilla casein or whey protein powder	No Change
¼ cup unsweetened raw shredded coconut	No Change

- Put into an electric blender the pears, coconut milk, almond meal, flaxseed, and casein or whey powder.
- Blend on low speed until the ingredients are completely combined and there are no large chunks of pear, but the mixture has a coarse texture.
- Add the coconut and blend just until the coconut is incorporated.
- Serve immediately.

German Chocolate Pancakes

Makes 2 servings

SANE	SANEst
6 egg whites	No Change
2 eggs	No Change
1 cup water	No Change
1 cup nonfat Greek yogurt	No Change
1 cup chocolate protein powder blend (I use UMP)	No Change
½ cup unsweetened raw shredded coconut	No Change
1 cup raw unsweetened cocoa powder (not dutch-processed)	No Change
6 tbsp Xyla xylitol	No Change
Cinnamon, to taste	No Change
Coconut oil spray	No Change

- Put all the ingredients except the coconut oil spray into a blender in the order listed.
- Blend on high until the mixture is completely smooth.
- Spray a skillet with coconut oil and place over medium heat.
- Heat the skillet for 2 minutes and pour the batter into the skillet.
- Cook for 2 to 3 minutes. Gently lift the edge of the pancake with a spatula to check for browning. Once the underside is lightly browned, flip the pancake and cook for 20 to 30 seconds until cooked all the way through.
- Serve immediately.

Grain-Free Granola

Makes 8 servings

SANE	SANEst
1 cup cashews, roughly chopped	½ cup cashews, roughly chopped
1 cup hazelnuts, roughly chopped	½ cup hazelnuts, roughly chopped
1 cup slivered almonds	1 cup slivered almonds
1 cup unsweetened shredded coconut	2 cups unsweetened shredded coconut
8 tbsp whole flaxseed	8 tbsp whole flaxseed
6 tsp ground nutmeg	6 tsp ground nutmeg
⅔ cup sugar-free vanilla syrup (such as Torani's)	⅔ cup sugar-free vanilla syrup (such as Torani's)
2 tbsp melted coconut oil	2 tbsp melted coconut oil

- Preheat the oven to 300°F.
- In a large bowl, mix the nuts, coconut, flaxseed, and nutmeg until combined.
- Add the syrup and oil and mix well, ensuring that the ingredients are evenly coated.
- On a foil-covered baking sheet, spread the mixture evenly in a half-inch layer.
- Bake on the middle rack of the oven until deep golden brown, stirring occasionally to ensure even coloring.
- Cool completely. Store in an airtight jar.

Ham and Eggs Bake

Makes 2 servings

SANE	SANEst
1 tbsp butter	½ tbsp coconut oil
6 tbsp heavy cream	n/a
4 oz cubed ham	6 oz cubed ham
2 tsp dried parsley	2 tsp dried parsley
Salt and freshly ground pepper	Salt and freshly ground pepper
4 eggs	4 eggs

- Preheat the oven to 350°F.
- Grease 2 small ramekins with the butter or oil.
- Pour 2 tbsp of the cream (if using) into the bottom of each ramekin.
- Spread the ham in the bottom of the ramekins and season with parsley and salt and pepper to taste.
- Carefully crack 2 eggs into each ramekin over the ham.
- Pour 1 tbsp of cream (if using) over the eggs in each ramekin.
- Place the ramekins in a small baking dish. Add warm water to the dish to come halfway up the side of the ramekins.
- Bake for 15 minutes, or until the eggs are just cooked through.

Pancakes

Makes 2 servings

SANE	SANEst
½ tsp pure vanilla extract	No Change
4 egg whites	No Change

2 eggs	No Change
1 cup nonfat Greek yogurt	No Change
½ cup water	No Change
1 cup vanilla UMP protein powder blend	No Change
½ cup unsweetened raw shredded coconut	No Change
Cinnamon, to taste	No Change
Fresh berries of your choice	No Change
Optional: sugar-free vanilla syrup, to serve	No Change
Coconut oil spray	No Change

- Place all the ingredients except the syrup in a blender in the order listed.
- Blend on high until the mixture is completely smooth.
- Lightly spray a large skillet with coconut oil and place over medium heat.
- Pour the batter into the hot skillet. Cook for 2 to 3 minutes. Gently lift the edge of the pancake to check for browning. Once the underside is lightly browned, flip the pancake and cook for 20 to 30 seconds on the other side.
- Serve immediately with fresh berries and syrup on top, if desired.

Super Yogurt

Makes 2 servings

SANE	SANEst
2 cups low-fat Greek yogurt	No Change
⅔ cup vanilla casein or whey powder	No Change
⅔ cup walnuts, chopped	No Change
Cinnamon, to taste	No Change

- Place all the ingredients in a bowl and mix well.
- Serve immediately.

Strawberry–Chia Seed Cereal

Makes 4 servings

SANE	SANEst
1⅓ cups light coconut milk	1¾ cups water
⅓ cup chia seeds	⅓ cup chia seeds

1 lb nonfat Greek yogurt	1 lb nonfat Greek yogurt
½ lb frozen strawberries	¼ lb frozen strawberries
	⅔ cup strawberry casein or whey powder

- Pour the coconut milk (or water) into a large bowl.
- Add the chia seeds and stir immediately to stop the seeds from sticking together.
- Add the yogurt and mix well. Add the frozen strawberries.
- Cover and refrigerate overnight.
- In the morning, add casein or whey powder (if using) and mix well until completely combined.
- Serve immediately.

Vanilla Almond Hot Cereal

Makes 2 servings

SANE	SANEst
2 tbsp chia seeds	2 tbsp chia seeds
2 tbsp sunflower seeds	1 tbsp sunflower seeds
4 tbsp unsweetened shredded coconut	7 tbsp unsweetened shredded coconut
2 tbsp ground flaxseed	2 tbsp ground flaxseed
4 tbsp almond meal	2 tbsp almond meal
2 tsp cinnamon	2 tsp cinnamon
⅔ cup vanilla casein or whey powder	⅔ cup vanilla casein or whey powder
1 cup boiling water	1 cup boiling water
½ tsp pure vanilla extract	½ tsp pure vanilla extract
2 tsp Xyla xylitol, or to taste	2 tsp Xyla xylitol, or to taste
2 oz fresh berries	2 oz fresh berries

- Place the chia seeds, sunflower seeds, and coconut in a coffee grinder and grind to a fine meal. Take care not to overgrind to a paste.
- Pour the ground mixture into a bowl. Add the flaxseed, almond meal, cinnamon, and casein or whey powder. Mix well until completely blended.
- Add the boiling water and mix well. Set aside for 1 minute to thicken.
- Mix again, adding more boiling water if you prefer a runnier cereal.
- Add the vanilla and xylitol to taste.
- Serve with the berries.

Strawberry-Avocado Green Smoothie

Makes 1 serving

SANE	SANEst
1 cup light coconut milk	1 cup coconut milk
4 cups fresh spinach	6 cups fresh spinach
1 small avocado, peeled and roughly chopped	1 small avocado, peeled and roughly chopped
⅔ cup strawberry casein or whey powder	½ cup (2 scoops) strawberry casein or whey powder
1 cup frozen strawberries	½ cup frozen strawberries
1 cup boiling water	1 cup boiling water

- Place all ingredients in a blender in the order listed.
- Blend on high until completely smooth.
- Serve immediately.

Orange Creamsicle Green Smoothie

Makes 1 serving

SANE	SANEst
½ cup coconut milk	½ cup coconut milk
¼ cup nonfat Greek yogurt	¼ cup nonfat Greek yogurt
6 cups fresh spinach	8 cups fresh spinach
2 peeled oranges	2 peeled oranges
Zest of ½ orange, chopped	Zest of ½ orange, chopped
1 cup vanilla casein or whey powder	1 cup vanilla casein or whey powder
½ tsp pure vanilla extract	½ tsp pure vanilla extract
½ tsp guar gum	½ tsp guar gum

- Place all ingredients except the guar gum in a blender in the order listed.
- Blend on high until completely smooth.
- Remove the blender lid stopper. While the blender is still running, shake the guar gum in.
- Blend for 10 seconds more (but no longer).
- Serve immediately.

Lunches

Broccoli and Red Pepper Miniquiches

Makes 3 servings

SANE	SANEst
3 oz red pepper, finely chopped	4 oz red pepper, finely chopped
4 oz broccoli, chopped	5 oz broccoli, chopped
2 oz sharp Cheddar, grated	6 oz nonfat cottage cheese
10 eggs	11 egg whites
1 tsp dried parsley	1 tsp dried parsley
¼ cup 2% Greek yogurt	n/a
Freshly ground pepper	Freshly ground pepper

- Preheat the oven to 375°F.
- Place 12 silicone baking cups in a muffin pan.
- In a large bowl, mix the red pepper, broccoli, and Cheddar or cottage cheese until well combined.
- Divide the vegetable mixture evenly among the 12 cups.
- Place the eggs (or whites), parsley, Greek yogurt (if using), and pepper to taste in a bowl and whisk well to combine. Pour the egg mixture into a pitcher.
- Carefully pour the egg mixture over the cheese mixture in each cup till almost full.
- Carefully place the muffin pan on the middle rack of the oven.
- Bake for 30 minutes (35 or more minutes for SANEst recipe) until puffy and golden brown, and a skewer comes out clean. The quiches will rise well above the cups.
- Remove the pan from the oven and carefully remove each quiche from its cup.
- Serve immediately.

Note: If you wish to make these in advance, allow the quiches to cool completely and store in an airtight container in the refrigerator.

Creamy Cucumber Soup

Makes 6 servings

SANE	SANEst
2 tbsp coconut oil	2 tbsp coconut oil
1 medium onion, chopped	1 medium onion, chopped

3 large English cucumbers, chopped	3 large English cucumbers, chopped
1½ cups light coconut milk	1½ cups water
1 tbsp salt	1 tbsp salt
½ cup chopped chives	½ cup chopped chives
2 small avocados, peeled and roughly chopped	2 small avocados, peeled and roughly chopped
2 tbsp heavy cream	2 tbsp 2% Greek yogurt
1 tbsp white wine	n/a

- In a large stockpot, melt the coconut oil over medium heat. Add the onion and sauté until transparent.
- Add the cucumber, coconut milk (or water), and salt, and cover the pot. Cook until the cucumber is tender, about 10 minutes. Remove from the heat.
- Working in batches, carefully transfer the cucumber mixture to a blender and blend on high until very smooth.
- To the last batch, add the chives, avocado, cream or yogurt, and white wine, if using. Blend until completely incorporated.
- Return the blended soup to the stockpot and stir well. Gently rewarm over low heat if necessary.
- Serve immediately.

Chicken, Avocado, and Walnut Salad

Makes 4 servings

SANE	SANEst
2 heads romaine lettuce	No Change
4 tbsp extra virgin olive oil	No Change
1½ tbsp Xyla xylitol	No Change
2 tbsp white wine vinegar	No Change
1 tbsp chopped parsley	No Change
¼ tsp dried oregano	No Change
Salt and freshly ground pepper	No Change
2 avocados	No Change
2 oz walnuts, roughly chopped	No Change
1 lb cooked chicken breast, cut into bite-size chunks	No Change

- Tear the lettuce into large pieces and place on a large serving dish.
- Whisk the olive oil, xylitol, vinegar, parsley, and oregano in a small bowl until completely blended. Season with salt and pepper to taste.
- Peel, halve, and slice the avocados.
- Add the avocados to the dressing and carefully turn to coat each slice.
- Spoon the avocados evenly over the bed of lettuce.
- Sprinkle the walnuts and chicken evenly over the salad.
- Drizzle the remaining dressing over the salad.
- Serve immediately.

Leek and Cauliflower Soup

Makes 6 servings

SANE	SANEst
4 cups chicken stock	5 cups chicken stock
¾ cup white cooking wine*	n/a
2 lbs thinly sliced leeks	2 lbs thinly sliced leeks
1 medium cauliflower, cut into small pieces	1 medium cauliflower, cut into small pieces
1 tsp dried rosemary	1 tsp dried rosemary
2 tsp dried mint	2 tsp dried mint
1 tsp salt	1 tsp salt
¼ cup melted butter	n/a

- Pour the stock and (if using) the wine into a large stockpot and place over medium heat.
- Add the leeks, cauliflower, rosemary, mint, and salt.
- Cover and cook until the cauliflower is just tender, about 15 minutes.
- Working in batches, put the vegetable mixture in a blender and blend on high until completely smooth. Add the butter (if using) to the last batch.
- Return the blended vegetables to the stockpot and stir well.

* Calories provided by the vast majority of alcoholic beverages are inSANE. That doesn't mean we must avoid all alcoholic beverages. It means that given our goal of minimizing inSANE calories, the best alcoholic beverages are those with the least calories. For example, choose wine instead of beer, choose clear liquor versus brown liquor, and completely avoid sugar-saturated mixers (for example, fruit juice or soda).

- Gently reheat if necessary.
- Serve immediately.

Peanut Butter–Chicken Salad

Makes 4 servings

SANE	SANEst
1 tbsp coconut oil	No Change
2 lbs chicken breasts sliced into small strips	No Change
4 medium carrots, peeled and sliced into thin sticks	No Change
1 large English cucumber, sliced into thin sticks	No Change
8 green onions (scallions), thinly sliced	No Change
1 lb bean sprouts, rinsed and drained well	No Change
6 oz salted roasted peanuts, roughly chopped	No Change
¼ cup natural crunchy peanut butter	No Change
½ cup chicken stock	No Change
4 tsp soy sauce	No Change
4 tbsp extra virgin olive oil	No Change
Freshly ground pepper	No Change
5 handfuls fresh baby spinach	No Change

- In a large skillet over medium heat, melt the coconut oil. Add the chicken strips and sauté until golden brown.
- Remove the chicken strips from the skillet and drain. Set aside to cool.
- Place the carrots, cucumber, onions, and bean sprouts in a large bowl.
- Add 4 oz of the peanuts.
- In a small bowl, whisk the peanut butter with the chicken stock and soy sauce.
- Slowly add the olive oil, whisking well until completely incorporated.
- Season with pepper to taste.
- Pour the peanut sauce over the vegetables and add the cooled chicken strips.
- Toss the ingredients until well coated in the sauce.
- Place the spinach on 4 plates; spoon a quarter of the chicken mixture onto each plate.
- Sprinkle the remaining 2 oz of peanuts over the salads.
- Serve immediately.

Smoked Salmon and Bean Sprout Sauté

Makes 2 servings

SANE	SANEst
2 tbsp coconut oil	No Change
1 lb leeks, thinly sliced	No Change
5 oz smoked salmon (lox), sliced into thin strips	No Change
½ cup 2% Greek yogurt	No Change
Freshly ground pepper	No Change
4 oz bean sprouts	No Change

- In a large skillet, melt the coconut oil over medium heat.
- Add the leeks and sauté until soft, about 10 minutes. Do not allow them to brown.
- Add the smoked salmon and yogurt; stir well.
- Add the bean sprouts and stir until evenly distributed through the mixture.
- Cook just long enough to warm through, about 2 minutes.
- Season with freshly ground pepper and serve immediately.

Dinners

Chicken Carbonara

Makes 4 servings

SANE	SANEst
2 tbsp coconut oil	2 tbsp coconut oil
1½ lbs chicken breast, cut into thin strips	2 lbs chicken breast, cut into thin strips
8 oz uncooked bacon slices, chopped	8 oz uncooked bacon slices, chopped
3 lbs Napa cabbage, shredded	3 lbs Napa cabbage, shredded
4 eggs	4 eggs
½ cup heavy cream	½ cup almond milk
Salt and freshly ground pepper	Salt and freshly ground pepper

- In a large skillet, heat the coconut oil over medium heat until melted. Preheat the broiler to 500°F.
- Sauté the chicken strips in the skillet until golden brown.
- Remove the chicken with a slotted spoon and place in an ovenproof serving dish. Cover with foil to keep warm.

- Add the bacon to the skillet and cook until crisp.
- Add the cabbage to the skillet and stir-fry with the bacon for two minutes, turning frequently.
- In a small bowl, beat together the eggs and cream (or almond milk). Season with salt and pepper to taste.
- Reduce the heat to its lowest setting. Add the egg mixture to the bacon and cabbage mixture.
- Stir constantly until well mixed and the egg mixture thickens, about 2 to 3 minutes.
- Stir in the chicken strips. Spoon the mixture into the ovenproof serving dish.
- Broil until the top bubbles and turns golden brown, 2 to 3 minutes.
- Serve immediately.

Lasagna

Makes 8 servings

SANE	SANEst
2 medium eggplants, cut lengthwise into ¼-inch slices	2 medium eggplants, cut lengthwise into ¼-inch slices
2 tbsp melted coconut oil	2 tbsp melted coconut oil
Freshly ground pepper	Freshly ground pepper
2 lbs grass-fed ground beef or turkey	2 lbs grass-fed ground beef or turkey
1 large jar (1 lb 8 oz) all-natural tomato basil sauce (no sugar added)	1 large jar (1 lb 8 oz) all-natural tomato basil sauce (no sugar added)
1 tsp xanthan gum	1 tsp xanthan gum
n/a	6 handfuls fresh spinach
1 lb 2% cottage cheese	1 lb nonfat cottage cheese
12 oz shredded mozzarella	8 oz shredded mozzarella
½ cup Parmesan, finely grated	n/a

- Preheat the oven to 400°F.
- Brush the eggplant slices with oil and season with pepper to taste. Place on foil-covered baking sheets.
- Bake for 20 minutes, turning eggplant slices after 10 minutes.
- Reduce the oven temperature to 375°F.
- In a large skillet over medium-high heat, brown the beef or turkey.
- Add the tomato sauce to the skillet, reduce the heat to low, and simmer uncovered for 20 minutes.

- While quickly stirring the meat sauce, sprinkle the xanthan gum over the surface and combine well.
- Spread ½ cup of the meat sauce on the bottom of a large baking dish.
- Place 6 slices of the eggplant to cover the bottom of the dish. Layer on half of the spinach, if using.
- Spread half of the remaining meat sauce over the eggplant.
- Spread half of the cottage cheese over the meat sauce.
- Spread half of the mozzarella over the cottage cheese.
- Place the remaining eggplant on top of the mozzarella to cover it. Layer on the remaining spinach, if using.
- Repeat the layers with the remaining meat sauce, cottage cheese, and mozzarella.
- Evenly sprinkle the Parmesan (if using) on top of the mozzarella.
- Bake for 20 minutes, rotating the dish after 10 minutes, or until the top is golden and bubbling.
- Serve immediately.

Pork Chops with Bacon and Cabbage

Makes 4 servings

SANE	SANEst
2 tbsp coconut oil	2 tbsp coconut oil
4 large pork chops	4 large pork chops
Salt and freshly ground pepper	Salt and freshly ground pepper
1 head green cabbage (2½ lbs), cut into 8 wedges	1 head green cabbage (2½ lbs), cut into 8 wedges
8 strips bacon, sliced into ½-inch pieces	4 strips bacon, sliced into ½-inch pieces
1 medium onion, chopped	1 medium onion, chopped
2 tbsp garbanzo bean flour	2 tbsp garbanzo bean flour
3 cups light coconut milk	3 cups chicken stock

- Preheat the oven to 400°F.
- Set a large, heavy roasting pan across two burners over medium heat. Add the oil and melt.
- Season the pork chops with salt and pepper to taste. Place in the pan and brown on one side, about 3 to 5 minutes. Turn and brown the other side. Transfer to a plate.

- Place the cabbage wedges, cut side down, in the roasting pan and cook until lightly browned, about 6 minutes. Turn and cook until slightly tender, about 3 minutes. Transfer to the plate with the pork chops.
- Place the bacon in the pan. Cook until golden, about 5 minutes. Add the onion and cook until softened, about 5 minutes.
- In a small bowl, mix the garbanzo bean flour with a tablespoon of the milk (or stock) to make a smooth, thin paste.
- Add the remaining milk (or stock) to the pan with the bacon and onions.
- Add the garbanzo bean paste to the milk in the pan. Stir the sauce constantly until thickened, about 4 minutes.
- Season the mixture with salt and pepper to taste, then return the pork chops and cabbage to the roasting pan.
- Transfer the pan to the middle rack of the oven.
- Bake until the pork is cooked through, about 10 minutes, and the sauce is bubbling and golden brown. If using thick bone-in chops, cook for about 15 minutes.

Prawn and Mushroom Stir-Fry

Makes 2 servings

SANE	SANEst
1 tbsp coconut oil	No Change
1 large leek, sliced	No Change
4 oz mushrooms, sliced	No Change
12 oz cooked prawns, tails removed	No Change
⅓ cup 2% Greek yogurt	No Change
Juice of half a lemon (about 2 tbsp)	No Change
Lemon pepper, sugar-free seasoning	No Change

- In a large skillet, melt the coconut oil over medium heat.
- Add the leek and sauté gently, stirring often, for 5 minutes or until tender.
- Add the sliced mushrooms. Cook for 1 minute.
- Add the prawns and cook just to heat through, about 2 minutes.
- Add the yogurt and toss with the prawn mixture until evenly coated.
- Stir in the lemon juice.
- Season liberally with lemon pepper.
- Serve immediately.

Salmon with Orange and Fennel

Makes 4 servings

SANE	SANEst
2 large oranges, peeled and segmented, juice reserved	No Change
1 small fennel bulb, very thinly sliced	No Change
¼ cup pitted green olives, halved	No Change
2 tbsp fresh lemon juice	No Change
1 tsp olive oil	No Change
Kosher salt and freshly ground pepper	No Change
2 tsp coconut oil	No Change
4 skinless salmon fillets	No Change

- In a bowl, combine the orange segments, reserved juice, fennel, olives, lemon juice, and olive oil. Season with salt and pepper to taste, toss gently, and set aside.
- In a large nonstick skillet, melt the coconut oil over medium heat.
- Add the salmon fillets, flat side down, and cook until browned, about 3 minutes.
- Turn and cook until opaque throughout, 1 to 3 minutes more, depending on thickness.
- Place the salmon fillets in a serving dish and spoon the orange mixture over each piece.
- Serve immediately.

Turkey and Almond Stir-Fry

Makes 2 servings

SANE	SANEst
1 tbsp coconut oil	No Change
6 oz broccoli-carrot slaw	No Change
⅓ cup slivered almonds	No Change
7 oz fresh smoked deli turkey, cut into strips	No Change
1 tsp dried rosemary	No Change
¼ cup 2% Greek yogurt	No Change
1 tbsp balsamic vinegar	No Change
Salt and freshly ground pepper	No Change

- In a large skillet, melt the coconut oil over high heat until steam starts to rise.
- Add the broccoli-carrot slaw and almonds. Stir-fry for 2 minutes, stirring constantly.

- Reduce the heat to medium.
- Add the turkey, stir, and cook for 1 minute.
- Add the rosemary and gently stir in the yogurt.
- Add the balsamic vinegar and stir well. Season with salt and pepper to taste.
- Serve immediately.

Turkey and Mushroom Stroganoff

Makes 4 servings

SANE	SANEst
2 lbs ground turkey or chicken	3 lbs ground turkey or chicken
8 oz mushrooms, sliced	8 oz mushrooms, sliced
2 cups chicken stock	4 cups chicken stock
1 cup fat-free milk	n/a
2 tbsp garbanzo bean flour	3 tbsp garbanzo bean flour
Salt and freshly ground pepper	Salt and freshly ground pepper
Dried oregano	Dried oregano
2 tbsp white wine vinegar	n/a

- In a large skillet over medium heat, brown the ground meat, stirring frequently to break it up.
- Add the mushrooms and cook for 1 minute.
- Add the chicken stock, stir well, and heat just until the mixture starts to bubble.
- Reduce the heat to low.
- In a small bowl, slowly mix the milk (or some stock from the skillet) into the garbanzo bean flour to make a thick paste.
- Add the paste to the meat mixture, stirring constantly until the sauce thickens.
- Simmer the meat sauce for 10 minutes.
- Season with salt, pepper, and oregano to taste. Add the vinegar, if using, and stir well.
- Serve the sauce spooned over piles of hot Squash Noodles (page 234).

Side Dishes

Almond Parmesan Squash

Makes 6 servings

SANE	SANEst
2 tbsp butter	2 tbsp coconut oil
2 lbs zucchini, cut into ¼-inch-thick slices	2 lbs zucchini, cut into ¼-inch-thick slices
1 medium onion, coarsely chopped	1 medium onion, coarsely chopped
Salt and freshly ground pepper	Salt and freshly ground pepper
¾ cup heavy cream	½ cup 2% Greek yogurt mixed with ¼ cup almond milk
½ cup almond meal, plus more for garnish	¼ cup almond meal, plus more for garnish
½ cup grated Parmesan, plus more for garnish	¼ cup grated Parmesan, plus more for garnish

- Preheat the oven to 450°F.
- In a large skillet, heat the butter or coconut oil over medium heat until melted.
- Add the zucchini and onion and season with salt and pepper to taste. Sauté, turning occasionally, until the vegetables are crisp-tender, about 5 minutes.
- Pour the cream or yogurt mixture over the vegetables and stir gently.
- Cook until thickened, about 5 minutes.
- Remove the skillet from the heat and gently stir in the almond meal, and then the Parmesan.
- Spoon the vegetable mixture into a baking dish.
- Sprinkle additional almond meal and Parmesan evenly over the mixture.
- Bake on the middle rack of the oven for 10 minutes until the top is golden brown.
- Serve immediately.

Squash Noodles

Makes 4 servings

SANE	SANEst
1 tbsp coconut oil	No Change
1 large leek, very thinly sliced	No Change

| 4 large yellow (summer) squashes, julienned | No Change |
| 2 large zucchini, julienned | No Change |

- In a large stockpot, melt the coconut oil over medium heat.
- Add the leek and sauté, stirring frequently, until it wilts, about 3 minutes.
- Reduce the heat to low, add the squash and zucchini, and toss with the leek. Cook until the squash is warmed through, about 1 minute.
- Serve immediately.

Note: You can julienne vegetables with a julienne peeler or a mandoline.

Zucchini and Cherry Tomato Salad

Makes 4 servings

SANE	SANEst
8 oz cherry tomatoes, halved or quartered	No Change
¼ cup chopped raw walnuts	No Change
2 tbsp fresh basil, torn into small pieces	No Change
2 tbsp extra virgin olive oil	No Change
1 zucchini, sliced paper thin with a vegetable peeler or mandoline	No Change

- Mix the tomatoes, walnuts, basil, and oil in a bowl.
- Season with salt and pepper to taste and leave to stand for 20 minutes.
- Add the zucchini, toss, and garnish with basil.
- Serve immediately.

Desserts

Caramel-Orange-Spice Cashews

Makes 8 servings

SANE	SANEst
1 egg white	No Change
¼ cup Torani's sugar-free caramel syrup	No Change
1 tsp pure vanilla extract	No Change

½ tsp orange extract	No Change
1 lb cashews	No Change
½ tsp salt	No Change
3 tsp cinnamon	No Change
Zest of 2 oranges, finely chopped	No Change

- Preheat the oven to 350°F.
- In a large bowl, whisk the egg white, syrup, vanilla, and orange extract until frothy.
- Add the cashews and stir until the nuts are well coated.
- Add the salt, cinnamon, and orange zest and toss until the cashews are evenly coated.
- Spread the nuts out on a foil-covered baking sheet.
- Bake on the middle rack of the oven for 25 minutes, stirring every 5 minutes to separate, until the nuts are a deep golden brown.
- Cool completely. Store in an airtight jar at room temperature.

Chocolate-Covered Berry Cream

Makes 2 servings

SANE	SANEst
2 cups frozen mixed berries, thawed	No Change
4 tbsp unsweetened, undutched cocoa powder	No Change
2 cups nonfat Greek yogurt	No Change
4 tsp Xyla xylitol	No Change

- Place the berries in a bowl and sift the cocoa powder over them. Stir until completely coated.
- Stir in the yogurt and xylitol.
- Serve immediately or store in a lidded container in the refrigerator.

Chocolate–Peanut Butter Fudge

Makes 4 to 6 servings

SANE	SANEst
1 cup natural peanut butter	No Change
2 cups chocolate protein powder blend (I use UMP)	No Change
2 cups chocolate casein or whey powder	No Change
1 cup unsweetened, undutched cocoa powder	No Change

Cinnamon, to taste	No Change
Xyla xylitol, to taste (start with a teaspoon)	No Change
Water as needed, for consistency	No Change

- Place the peanut butter in a mixing bowl. Microwave for 30 seconds until it is softened.
- Add the remaining ingredients (except water) and mix well.
- Add water as needed to achieve the desired consistency.

Cinnamon-Raisin "Rice" Pudding

Makes 1 serving

SANE	SANEst
1 cup low-fat cottage cheese	1 cup nonfat cottage cheese
⅓ cup vanilla casein or whey powder	⅓ cup vanilla casein or whey powder
¼ cup raisins	n/a
1 tsp cinnamon	Cinnamon, to taste

- Place all the ingredients in a bowl and mix gently until combined.
- Serve immediately.

Note: For variety, substitute ½ cup Greek yogurt for ½ cup of the cottage cheese.

Dark Chocolate–Espresso Cookies

Makes 32 servings

SANE	SANEst
8 oz unsweetened 100% chocolate	No Change
¾ cup coconut oil	No Change
9 oz Xyla xylitol	No Change
2 eggs	No Change
1 tsp pure vanilla extract	No Change
6 oz almond flour	No Change
2 oz raw unsweetened, undutched cocoa powder	No Change
3 tsp instant espresso powder	No Change
2 tsp baking powder	No Change

½ tsp salt	No Change
1½ tsp xanthan gum	No Change
⅓ cup light coconut milk	No Change

- Preheat the oven to 325°F.
- Melt the chocolate in a heatproof bowl set over a pan of simmering water. Set aside to cool.
- In a large mixing bowl, beat the coconut oil and xylitol until they are completely blended and resemble very fine bread crumbs.
- Add the eggs and vanilla and beat until fully incorporated.
- Add the melted chocolate and stir until combined.
- In another bowl, whisk the almond flour, cocoa powder, espresso powder, baking powder, salt, and xanthan gum until combined. Add to the egg mixture and fold in until combined.
- Add the coconut milk and mix until combined.
- Roll 32 golf-ball-sized pieces of dough and place on foil-covered baking sheets, 2 inches apart. Flatten each ball into a disk ½ inch thick.
- Place the baking sheets on the middle rack of the oven and bake for 10 to 12 minutes. The cookies will look dry but will be still be soft in the center when they are done.
- Remove the cookies from the oven and leave on the baking sheet until cool to the touch. Carefully move the cookies to a rack to cool completely.
- Store in an airtight container.

Mint Chocolate Pudding

Makes 4 servings

SANE	SANEst
13 oz avocado flesh (3 small or 2 medium)	13 oz avocado flesh (3 small or 2 medium)
½ cup canned coconut cream	¾ cup light coconut milk
1 cup unsweetened, undutched cocoa powder	1 cup unsweetened, undutched cocoa powder
Pinch salt	Pinch salt
¼ tsp pure peppermint extract	¼ tsp pure peppermint extract
½ cup plus 3 tbsp Xyla xylitol	Xyla xylitol, to taste
n/a	⅓ cup chocolate casein or whey powder
2 tbsp cocoa nibs	2 tbsp cocoa nibs

- Place the avocado flesh and coconut cream or milk in a blender and blend on high until smooth.
- Add the cocoa powder, salt, peppermint extract, and xylitol and blend on high.
- Add the casein or whey powder, if using, and blend on low until completely mixed.
- Spoon into 4 glasses or dishes and refrigerate for at least 30 minutes until chilled.
- Sprinkle with the cocoa nibs and serve.

Note: You will need to stop the blender and stir the ingredients regularly, as this is very thick. It will be hard work for even the best blenders.

Orange-Cranberry Scones

Makes 8 servings

SANE	SANEst
9 oz almond flour	No Change
2 tbsp Xyla xylitol	No Change
2 tsp baking powder	No Change
1 tsp xanthan gum	No Change
½ tsp salt	No Change
2 oz (4 tbsp) butter	No Change
3 oz dried cranberries, chopped	No Change
Zest of 1 orange, finely chopped	No Change
1 egg, beaten	No Change
3 tbsp orange juice	No Change
1 additional egg, beaten, for brushing	No Change

- Preheat the oven to 425°F.
- Place the almond flour, xylitol, baking powder, xanthan gum, salt, and butter in a food processor and pulse the mixture resembles fine bread crumbs.
- Pour into a mixing bowl, add the cranberries and zest, and mix gently till combined.
- Beat the egg with the orange juice and add to the dry ingredients in the bowl.
- Mix just until a dough forms.
- Knead the dough lightly (2 or 3 turns) on an almond-floured surface.
- Roll out the dough to ½-inch thickness. Cut out 8 scones with a fluted cutter.
- Place scones 1 inch apart on a foil-covered baking sheet and brush with a beaten egg.
- Bake on the middle rack of the oven for 8 to 10 minutes or until golden brown.
- Serve warm.

Peanut Butter Mousse

Makes 6 servings

SANE	SANEst
2 cups nonfat Greek yogurt	No Change
1 cup natural peanut butter	No Change
1 cup vanilla casein or whey powder	No Change
3 egg whites	No Change
½ tsp cream of tartar	No Change
⅓ cup xylitol	

- In a large bowl, beat together the yogurt and peanut butter until completely blended.
- Mix in the casein or whey powder.
- In a separate bowl, beat the egg whites and cream of tartar until stiff.
- Add half of the xylitol and whisk in until well combined. Add the remaining xylitol and whisk until the egg whites are stiff and glossy.
- Gently fold the egg whites into the peanut butter mixture until completely blended.
- Spoon into 6 dishes and chill in the refrigerator before serving.

Your Smarter Exercise Program

The smarter exercise program can be summed up in seven words (inspired by Michael Pollan):

Exercise Forcefully. Not Too Often. Mostly Eccentric.

The smarter exercise program takes at most twenty minutes per week, so it cannot be complex. All it takes is four eccentric exercises performed for ten minutes, once per week, along with ten minutes of smarter interval training once per week (this can be done at home or at a gym). Please read Appendix A: To Do before Exercising Smarter (see page 276) before starting this program.

THE WEEKLY PROGRAM
- Day 1: 10 minutes of eccentric training
- Day 2: Relax and recover
- Day 3: Relax and recover
- Day 4: 10 minutes of smarter interval training
- Day 5: Relax and recover
- Day 6: Relax and recover
- Day 7: Relax and recover

After our discussion about needing a week to recover from eccentric exercise, you may be wondering why you would do both eccentric training and smarter interval training each week. Two smarter workouts per week make sense only for people new to smarter exercise because safety is most important and you need to ease your way into smarter exercise. Because of this it will take a while before you are able to safely use enough resistance to work your muscles completely. Since your most beneficial type 2b muscle fibers will not be getting exercised right from the start, two smarter workouts per week are fine. Once you are comfortable using the amount of resistance necessary to work all your muscle fibers, you can skip the smarter interval training.

Here is how you can tell when to cut back to one smarter workout per week:

1. Do eccentric training and write down the amount of resistance used. For example: "Did six eccentric shoulder presses with 20 pounds."
2. Rest for two days.
3. Do smarter interval training.
4. Rest for three days.
5. Do eccentric training with the same resistance used last time.

If steps three and five are possible, you are not exercising your type 2b muscle fibers yet (that is, you are not using enough resistance for your eccentric shoulder press) and should stick with two smarter workouts per week until you are comfortable adding more resistance. If you were using enough resistance to activate your type 2b muscle fibers, your smarter interval training would have gone badly. Your still exhausted type 2b muscle fibers in your legs would not have worked well. If you somehow dragged your exhausted muscles through the smarter interval training, they would then be unable to meet the demands of eccentric training three days later.

TEN MINUTES OF ECCENTRIC TRAINING

If you are familiar with resistance training, you are familiar with sets and reps. If you are not familiar, you are better off because sets and reps are irrelevant. Muscle fibers do not care how many sets or reps we do. Dr. Ralph Carpinelli, of the Human Performance Laboratory at

Adelphi University, tells us, "There are fifty-seven studies . . . that show no statistically significant difference in the magnitude of strength gains or muscular [development] as a result of performing a greater number of sets."[181]

All our muscle fibers care about is how much force they need to generate. So let's focus on making as many muscle fibers as possible generate as much force as possible, doing whichever set of the following exercises we would like, once per week.*

Home Exercises	Gym Exercises
Eccentric Squats	Eccentric Leg Presses
Eccentric Pull-Ups	Eccentric Pull-Ups
Eccentric Push-Ups	Eccentric Chest Press
Eccentric Shoulder Press	Eccentric Shoulder Press

More exercises provide little if any value. You can think about doing more exercises to make your set-point lower just as you'd think about heating boiling water to make it hotter. In both cases we are just wasting energy.

Specific instructions on how to do these eccentric exercises are coming up. Also, most gyms will give you one free personal-training session in which you can ask the trainer to show you how to do the traditional versions of these exercises. On your own you can then apply the Six Principles of Smarter Exercise and be all set without spending any money. Best of all, there's no need to be intimidated. If you have ever sat down, opened a door, pushed something, or lifted anything above your head, you are most of the way to being an eccentric exercise expert.

Keep in mind that while the smarter workout is simple, it is not easy. We are trading quantity for quality and that is hard. For example, go back to the staircase you used earlier to see how much stronger you are eccentrically. Walk up it normally and note how you feel. Now wait

---

* Note: Both sets of exercises are basically the same. The gym options are performed on machines that enable us to add much more resistance safely. These machines are required for advanced individuals, as they will otherwise not be able to safely use the amount of resistance needed to activate all their muscle fibers.

a few minutes and walk up the same staircase two steps at a time. Notice how that is more tiring? In both cases you did the same quantity of exercise, but taking two steps at a time requires more force and works more muscle fibers.

Ten minutes of eccentric training should be like walking up a dozen stairs at a time. You will generate more force and work more muscle fibers than you ever did before. At the end of each exercise you will be exhausted. It will not be fun, but the results are incredible. Think of it as being like an immunization. You accept safe and short-term discomfort now to avoid life-threatening and long-term discomfort later. Plus, it is encouraging to know that you have to do it only once per week for ten minutes!

WHAT ABOUT MY ARMS AND ABS?

You do not need to do arm- and ab-specific exercises. If you enjoy doing them, that's fine, but please do them after the four eccentric exercises just listed and be sure they do not compromise your ability to perform those primary exercises.

Our goal is to work as much muscle as possible and arm- and ab-specific exercises work a little muscle. Besides, our four exercises work our arms and abs along with a bunch of other muscles, and the hormonal impact of these "big" exercises benefits our arms and abs more than biceps curls or crunches ever could.

In my favorite study of all time, researchers at the University of Southern Denmark divided people into two groups. The first group trained only one of their arms. The second group trained only one arm exactly the same way as the first group, but also trained both legs. With this creative setup, researchers could see what affected people's arm muscles more: direct arm training or the hormones triggered by all the muscle fibers worked using leg exercises. They could answer the following questions: How much stronger does an arm get if people

Do not train it?	[untrained arm + untrained legs]
Train only it?	[trained arm + untrained legs]
Do not train it, but do train their legs?	[untrained arm + trained legs]
Train it and train their legs?	[trained arm + trained legs]

Here are the results:

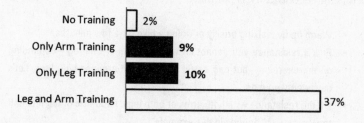

Clearly training legs along with arms is our best bet, but the fun part is the middle two bars. Resistance training only the legs increased *arm* strength more than resistance training only the arms. Why? Leg training worked more muscle and therefore triggered more whole-body-transforming hormones than arm training. All those hormones benefit seemingly unrelated muscles more than exercising those muscles directly. That is why we will work our biggest muscle groups (legs, back, chest, and shoulders) directly and our small muscle groups (arms, abs, etc.) indirectly. By focusing on the big things directly and the little things indirectly, we will take care of the little things better than we could any other way.

But seriously, what about our abdominal muscles? Don't we want a flat, toned tummy? Absolutely. But doing abdominal-only exercises before we lower our body fat percentage to the midteens is like worrying about how shiny a ring looks while wearing a boxing glove over it. The fastest way to "get abs" has nothing to do with exercising our abdominal muscles. We have to uncover our abdominal muscles—that is, unclog and lower our set-point.

Important Note: Make sure that you eat one of your at-least-30-gram servings of protein as soon as possible after your workouts. This aids in recovery and magnifies many of the metabolic benefits of smarter exercise. If you enjoy protein shakes, there is no better time to enjoy one than immediately after your workouts.

HOW TO EXERCISE ECCENTRICALLY

Exercising eccentrically is simple:

- Warm up by walking briskly or riding a bike for a few minutes.
- Pick a resistance you cannot lift with one arm or one leg—depending on the exercise—but can easily lift with both arms or both legs. Let's say twenty pounds.
- Lift the resistance with both arms or both legs. Each arm or leg lifts half the weight—10 pounds in this example.
- Lower the resistance with only one arm or one leg for ten seconds. Each arm or leg lowers all the weight—twenty pounds in our example—slowly.
- Repeat until it is impossible to lower the resistance with only one arm or one leg for ten seconds. If this takes more than six repetitions, gradually add resistance until it takes only six repetitions.

With this technique, you can exercise eccentrically in the comfort of your own home and bend many resistance-training machines at your local gym to your every eccentric whim. But before we get eccentric, there are two important rules to keep in mind.

First, if we choose to exercise eccentrically on resistance-training machines, then we should use only machines that work both of our arms or both of our legs *together*. This is the only way to have less resistance on the way up and more on the way down. If we pick machines that work our arms and legs independently, we will lift and lower the same amount of resistance. That defeats the whole purpose. Think about it this way. Say you grab a gallon of milk in each hand, lift both jugs above your head, and then drop the one in your right hand to increase the resistance for your left hand. That does not work because lifting milk jugs works your arms independently. However, if you lifted one milk jug with each arm, but then lowered both jugs with only your left arm, you would lower more resistance with your left arm than you lifted with your left arm. Resistance training machines that work both of our arms or both of our legs together do the same thing.

Second, exercise eccentrically only when *little, if any, balance is needed*. Just as you would not pick up a giant flat-screen TV with two hands and then let go with one, you should exercise eccentrically only when minimal balance is needed.

Let's put the two rules together. We could: Do a push-up with our knees on the floor (to reduce the resistance), and then lift our knees and lower ourselves (to increase the resistance). Our arms *work together* to lift a shared source of resistance (our body), and *little if any balance is needed*. Similarly, we could stand up and then do a body-weight squat down—while hanging on to something for balance—with one leg and then stand back up using both legs.

HOW TO EXERCISE ECCENTRICALLY AT HOME

Remember two key points when you start exercising eccentrically. First and foremost, nothing is more important than safety. The quickest way to compromise clog-clearing is to get hurt. Eccentric training is designed specifically to minimize injury—it is slow and controlled, it requires minimal balance, and you can spot yourself—but you still need to ease into it and to keep perfect form.

Second, once you have the hang of safely executing these exercises, you have to push yourself as hard as you safely can. You are trading quantity for quality, so it is particularly important that you maximize the quality of these exercises. If you do not, you will have thrown quantity and quality out the window. That is not exercising less—smarter. That is just exercising less.

Please push yourself as hard as you safely can and then continue to push yourself more and more by gradually adding resistance at least every other workout. As you improve the quality of your health and fitness, you must improve the quality of your exercise to keep progressing. Think about training your body as you would think about training your mind. Once we've mastered our multiplication tables, we have to move on to something more challenging to maximize our mental capacity. Same thing goes with our body. We have to keep adding resistance and challenging ourselves to maximize our physical capacity.

HOW TO INCREASE THE RESISTANCE OF AT-HOME ECCENTRICS

You can increase the effectiveness of your eccentric exercise in five safe ways, once you get the hang of it:

- Safely add resistance until it "lowers itself."
- Squat down lower.
- Hold the most challenging part of the movement.
- Buy resistance bands and a weight vest.
- Once you master at-home eccentrics, join an inexpensive gym.

Safely Add Resistance until It "Lowers Itself"

When you first start with eccentrics, you should consciously lower moderate resistance for ten seconds to get the hang of the movement. This will seem challenging, but not too bad. Once you feel that you have mastered the movement, add resistance and you will be surprised to see that you can still lower it for ten seconds. When you are completely comfortable with the movement, continue to add resistance until you no longer have to "try" to lower the resistance. You will do all that you can to stay still, but the correct level of resistance will force you down over the course of ten seconds.

Squat Down Lower

Squatting down four inches will not get us where we want to go, but we need to start somewhere. As we get stronger and more confident with the leg exercises we should increase our range of motion. For squats and leg presses, we gradually work our way to bending at the knee until our thighs are parallel with the ground (for squats) and platform (for leg presses) or a few inches lower.

Hold the Most Challenging Part of the Movement

For squats and leg presses, we squat down at a modest speed until our thighs are at least parallel with the ground/platform. We then hold that most challenging part of the movement for ten seconds rather than holding the top of the movement (the least challenging part of the movement) for most of the time.

Buy Resistance Bands and a Weight Vest

These are inexpensive substitutes for dumbbells and barbells at home. Put the weight vest on during your squats, pull-ups, and push-ups to increase resistance. Wrap the resistance bands around something sturdy and use them to increase the resistance of your shoulder presses.

Once You Master At-Home Eccentrics, Join an Inexpensive Gym

At some point you will get into such great shape that your body weight, resistance bands, and weight vests no longer provide enough resistance to work all your muscle fibers. At this point, if you want to improve your fitness, you'll need to use the machines at a gym.

Keep in mind that the most basic and inexpensive gym will do the trick. You need only the four machines outlined in the next section. Unless you are an elite athlete, protect yourself from the complexity that many gyms try to sell you. The more complex a gym tries to make exercise sound, the faster you should run in the other direction. Actual fitness experts know that 99 percent of the population can achieve all their goals using a leg-press type of movement, a pull-up or row movement, and chest- and shoulder-press movements. Everything else should be seen as "extended warranties." The person selling it to you will make it sound wondrous, but it is generally useless for everyone except the salesperson.

"How hard do I need to push myself to get *the best* results?" Think of effort as a scale of 1 to 10 where 1 is sleeping and 10 is giving birth. If your goals are ambitious, your effort needs to be ambitious. Aim for ten minutes per week of effort as close to level 10 as possible, always putting safety first. If your goal is more modest, your effort can be more modest too.

Eccentric Exercise How-To Videos

To get the most out of your eccentric exercises and interval training, check out the free how-to videos at www.SANESolution.com before you begin.

HOW TO EXERCISE ECCENTRICALLY AT HOME

Assisted Eccentric Squats

Muscle Groups Worked: Legs and Glutes

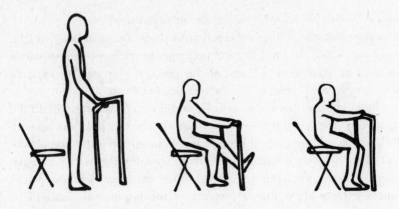

- Stand with your feet shoulder-width apart in front of something sturdy that you can hold on to with both hands. I use a railing or a doorknob. Put a chair behind you.
- Grab the sturdy thing in front of you and lean back until your arms are fully extended. Stand with all your weight on one of your heels. Make sure to keep your head and shoulders back while sticking your chest and butt out.
- Keeping all your weight on one of your heels, and keeping yourself balanced by holding on to that sturdy thing in front of you, sit down using only the one leg you put all your weight on. Use your non-weight-bearing leg to keep your balance and to ensure that you can lower yourself slowly and safely for ten seconds. If you can lower yourself for longer than ten seconds, then you are using your other leg too much. If you cannot lower yourself for ten seconds, then you are not using your other leg enough.
- Make sure that your knees never stick out farther than your toes while you are lowering yourself.
- Stop lowering yourself with one leg once your butt touches the chair. Keep holding on to the sturdy thing in front of you. Stand back up using both legs.
- Repeat this five more times and then do the same thing with your other leg.
- As you get stronger, remove the chair and try to squat down as far as you comfortably can without your heel lifting off the ground or your knees sticking out farther than your toes.

Assisted Eccentric Pull-Ups

Muscle Groups Worked: Back and Arms

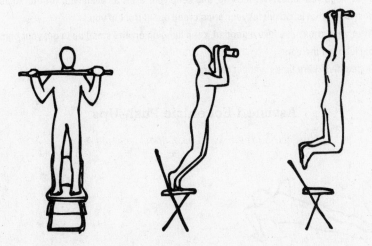

- Find something sturdy to hang from. It should be no lower than your chin if you are standing on the ground and no higher than your chin if you are standing on a chair. Common options include: jungle gyms/swing-sets, tree branches, or an inexpensive pull-up bar you've installed in your home.
- Stand on the ground or on a chair so that your chin is slightly above the thing you are going to hang from.
- With your arms slightly wider than shoulder-width apart, put your hands on top of the thing you are going to hang from. Grip it as tightly as you can. Stick your chest out and squeeze your shoulder blades together.
- With a firm grip, start to bend your legs so that you begin to hang from whatever it is you are holding on to. The more you bend your legs, the more challenging it will be to hang on.
- Bend your legs enough that you cannot hang on for longer than ten seconds. If you can hang on for longer than ten seconds, bend your legs more. If you cannot hang on for ten seconds, bend your legs less. Depending on your strength level, you may not need to use your legs at all.
- While you are hanging on, your back and arms will get tired and you will slowly lower down until your arms are fully extended. If your arms fully extend in less than

ten seconds, you are using your legs too little. If your arms fully extend in more than ten seconds, you are using your legs too much.

- While your arms are extending and you are lowering down, keep your shoulders back, keep your chest out, look up, and keep your arms as even with your torso as possible—that is, do not let your arms creep out in front of you.
- After your arms have fully extended, keep hanging on and stand up to get your chin back above the bar.
- Repeat five more times without resting.

Assisted Eccentric Push-Ups

Muscle Groups Worked: Chest, Shoulders, and Arms

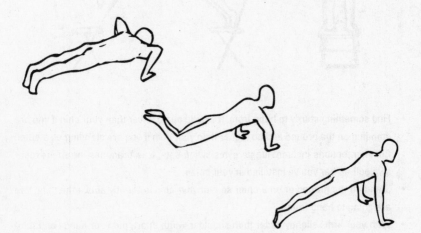

- Lie facedown on a clean floor and put your arms out to your sides so that your hands are even with your upper chest and slightly wider than shoulder-width apart.
- Keeping your knees on the floor, push yourself up through the palms of your hands until just before your elbows lock. You will now have only your knees and your hands touching the floor.
- Lift your knees off the floor and shift your weight to your toes. You will now have only your toes and hands touching the floor.
- With your shoulders back and your chest out, slowly lower yourself until just before any other part of your body touches the ground. Hold that position for ten sec-

onds. Make sure you keep your body in a straight line throughout the movement. Do not let your chest or hips bow down.

- After ten seconds, put your knees back on the floor and push yourself back up as you did originally. Once you have lowered yourself six times—for ten seconds each time, without resting in between times—you are done.
- If you cannot lower yourself six times—for ten seconds each time—put your knees back on the floor until you can.
- If you can lower yourself more than six times—for ten seconds each time—do not ever let your knees touch the floor. Always have just your hands and toes touching the floor. If that is still too easy, put your toes on something six to twelve inches off the ground. If that is still too easy, put your toes on something six to twelve inches off the ground and put something heavy on your back.

Assisted Eccentric Shoulder Press

Muscle Groups Worked: Shoulders and Arms

- Find something that you can safely lift above your head using both arms. You should also be able to safely hold it above your head with one arm. This means it should be small. Ideally you would use a dumbbell. Hold it in both hands.
- Lift it above your head using both hands. You should now be standing with your shoulders back and your chest out, holding something above your head with both arms extended as much as they can be without locking at the elbows.

- Very carefully release one hand but keep it close to whatever you are holding above your head to help lower it if needed.
- Keep the arm supporting the resistance to your side—that is, do not let it creep in front of you—and slowly lower the resistance for ten seconds, always keeping your other hand close by.
- If you can lower the resistance for more than ten seconds, you need something heavier. If you cannot lower the resistance for ten seconds, you need something lighter.
- Repeat this five more times—without resting—and then do the same thing with your other arm.

HOW TO EXERCISE ECCENTRICALLY AT A GYM

Before you get eccentric at your local gym, keep in mind that every brand of exercise machine is slightly different. Read the instructions on the machines you will be using to learn specifically how to lower the resistance, raise the resistance, position the seat, and position the handles.

Eccentric Leg Presses

Muscle Groups Worked: Legs and Glutes

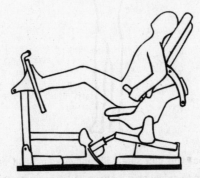

- Sit on the leg press machine with your back against the pad. Make sure to keep your head and shoulders back, while sticking your chest out. Think about how military personnel stand at attention. Do that with your head, shoulders, and back while sitting on the machine. This protects your back from injury. Never, ever, round your back forward during any exercise.

- Put your feet on the platform. Space your feet slightly wider than shoulder-width apart—whatever is most comfortable for you. Make sure your feet are high enough on the platform that your toes stay higher than your knees when you lower the resistance.
- When you lower and raise the resistance, make sure your knees stay lined up with your feet. Do not bow your legs in or out. Make sure your knees never stick out farther than your toes.
- Always push on the platform through your heels, while keeping your abs tight and your back against the pad, with your shoulders, back, and chest out.
- Lower the resistance for ten seconds with one leg, as low as you comfortably can without your back coming off the pad or your heels lifting off the platform.
- When you lift the resistance—with both legs—avoid locking your knees at the top of the movement. Right before you begin to lock your knees, start lowering the resistance with one leg again.
- Repeat this five more times—without resting—and then do the same thing with your other leg.

Eccentric Rows

Muscle Groups Worked: Back and Arms

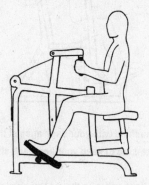

- Sit on the row machine and put your chest against the pad, if there is one. Either way, make sure to keep your back perpendicular to the floor with your head and shoulders back, while sticking your chest out. Imagine trying to pinch a playing card between your shoulder blades. Do that with your back and shoulders while you lift and lower the resistance.

- Put your feet flat on the floor or flat on the machine's platform. Keep them there.
- When you lift and lower the resistance, keep your torso still. Use only your back and arm muscles to lift the resistance. Do not move your torso to generate momentum to help your back and arms.
- Lift with both arms, then lower the resistance for ten seconds with one arm until your arm extends as far as it can, without causing you to round your back or to lock your elbow. Repeat "shoulders back, chest out" in your mind during this and all other exercises.
- Just before your elbow begins to lock, use both arms to lift the resistance again.
- Repeat this five more times—without resting—and then do the same thing with your other arm.

Eccentric Chest Press

Muscle Groups Worked: Chest, Shoulders, and Arms

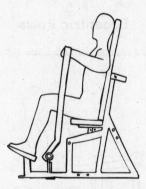

- Sit on the chest press machine with your back against the pad, as you did with the leg press machine. Make sure to keep your head and shoulders back, while sticking your chest out.
- Put your feet flat on the floor or flat on the machine's platform. Keep them there.
- When you lower and lift the resistance, make sure you keep your shoulders and head back, abs tight, and chest out. Do not lift your lower back off the pad.
- When you lift the resistance with both arms, extend your arms as far as they will

go without locking your elbows or moving your shoulders forward. Just before your elbows begin to lock, start slowly lowering the resistance.

- Lower the resistance for ten seconds with one arm until your hand is about even with your rib cage.
- Repeat this five more times—without resting—and then do the same thing with your other arm.

Eccentric Shoulder Press

Muscle Groups Worked: Shoulders and Arms

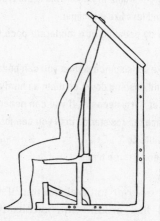

- Sit on the shoulder press machine with your back against the pad as you did with the chest press machine. Make sure to keep your head and shoulders back, while sticking your chest out.
- Put your feet flat on the floor or flat on the machine's platform. Keep them there.
- When you lower and lift the resistance, make sure you keep your shoulders and head back, abs tight, and chest out. Do not lift your lower back off the pad.
- When you lift the resistance with both arms, extend your arms as far as they will go without locking your elbows or moving your shoulders up. Just before your elbows begin to lock, start slowly lowering the resistance.
- Lower the resistance for ten seconds with one arm until your hand is about even with your shoulders.
- Repeat this five more times—without resting—and then do the same thing with your other arm.

HOW TO DO SMARTER INTERVAL TRAINING

> The efficacy of a high intensity exercise protocol, involving only
> ~250 kcal [calories] of work each week, to substantially improve
> insulin action [unclog] in young sedentary subjects is remarkable.
>
> —Dr. John Babraj, Heriot-Watt University[182]

Since you already know how to pedal on an upright stationary bike
you are ready for smarter interval training:

1. Hop onto an upright stationary bike. This is the type that looks more like a regular bike and less like a recliner.
2. Get warmed up by pedaling at a moderate pace with moderate resistance.
3. Increase the bike's resistance so that you can pedal only by standing up on the pedals and pushing down on them as hard as you can.
4. Pedal like that for thirty seconds. If you can pedal for longer than thirty seconds, increase the resistance until you cannot.
5. Rest for two minutes.
6. Repeat steps 4 and 5 three times.

We're not doing *smarter* interval training if we get on an upright
stationary bike and flail around uncontrollably for thirty seconds.
Sounds silly, but that is exactly what will happen if we don't add a lot
of resistance. Assuming you are not a highly trained athlete—moving
your body very quickly will eventually lead to an injury. However, after
you add resistance, you can move at a normal, controllable, and safe
rate, while working as forcefully as you possibly can. As a general rule
of thumb, *smarter* interval training is not about moving faster. It's about
moving more resistance.

Keep in mind that you don't have to use an upright stationary bike,
but you do need to use a low-impact machine that will provide you
with enough resistance to exhaust yourself in thirty seconds without
having to move quickly. This means you cannot do smarter cardio on a
treadmill, as that would be extremely high impact and there is no way
to safely add sufficient resistance.

Home Option		Add resistance?
Assisted Eccentric Squats	Resistance: _____	Y / N
Assisted Eccentric Pull-Ups	Resistance: _____	Y / N
Assisted Eccentric Push-Ups	Resistance: _____	Y / N
Assisted Eccentric Shoulder Press	Resistance: _____	Y / N
Gym Option		Add resistance?
Eccentric Squats	Resistance: _____	Y / N
Eccentric Pull-Ups	Resistance: _____	Y / N
Eccentric Chest Press	Resistance: _____	Y / N
Eccentric Shoulder Press	Resistance: _____	Y / N
		Add resistance?
10 Minutes of Smarter Interval Training	Resistance: _____	Y / N

Remember, for eccentric training, start slow and add resistance once you can lower the resistance you have now for ten seconds more than six times. As a general rule, you will know you have arrived at the right resistance and intensity levels when you stop questioning how this one workout per week leads to lasting fat loss and start questioning how you will walk upstairs for the rest of the week given how sore you are.

For smarter interval training, add resistance once you can pedal against the resistance level for more than thirty seconds at a time.

Finally, if someone tells you that you must do different exercises to see results, that person does not have all the facts. It is 100 percent true that we must continue to challenge our muscles if we want to continue to improve. However, this is most effectively done by adding resistance, not by adding complexity.

Conclusion:
Fight Fat with Facts

True scientists put the solution to a medical problem first and not the preservation of their own hypothesis, no matter how clever the hypothesis may seem or how proud of themselves they may be for creating it.

—Uffe Ravnskov, MD, PhD[183]

If two billion people can be selective about what they eat, so can we. Take the dietary restrictions of the Islamic, Hindu, and Jewish religions; add diabetics and vegetarians; assume a third of these people skip the restrictions; and we end up with about two billion people worldwide who eat in a way that is much tougher than SANEity. These billions of people are not "better" than we are. We too can be intentional about what we put into our bodies. Also, most people spend an average of over twenty-four minutes per day driving to and from work. Everyone has ten to twenty minutes *per week* to spend driving hormonal clogs from the body via eccentric exercise. We have all done more difficult and less beneficial things than eating more and exercising less—but smarter. Now, armed with the right information, we have the ability to feel better and burn body fat forever.

As you start seeing dramatic improvements in your health, appearance, energy levels, and mood, people will ask questions that mask their envy. "Don't you like food?" is a common remark. Our lifestyle is the opposite of disliking food. We are eating more food. Our disapproving peers are the ones trying to eat less of it. Sure, we are selective about what we eat, but to say that means we dislike food is like saying that being selective about what we listen to means we dislike music. Just remember Dr. Seuss's timeless advice: "Those who mind do not matter and those who matter do not mind."

Beyond specific food-related jabs, the envious will generally try to bring you back to "normal." The best way to deal with the constant coaxing is to keep some simple logic in mind: if you do not want what everyone else has, you should not do what everyone else does. Put differently: if you do not want typical results, you should not do what is typically done.

As we have seen throughout this book, our approach is based on scientific findings, not on opinion. It is not an opinion that our body regulates our weight automatically. Calories do have different qualities. Hormones are important. Starches are more harmful than helpful. Added sweeteners are addictive and toxic. Protein and fat are essential while carbohydrate is not. Nonstarchy vegetables, nutrient-dense protein, whole-food fats, and low-fructose fruits are the SANEst foods. And it is not an opinion that we get better results more safely by exercising more muscle slowly.

Let's review the key points of our SANE Solution:

- Telling hormonally clogged people to eat less and exercise more is like telling depressed people to frown less and smile more. Both cases confuse temporarily suppressing symptoms with addressing the underlying issue: *low-quality* inputs.
- Our set-point automatically regulates our body fat levels long term. Chronic body fat gain is the result of a hormonal clog that raises our set-point.
- Long-term fat loss and health come from clearing this clog and lowering our set-point. Long-term fat loss comes from making our body work like the bodies of people who eat whatever they want and do not get fat. Long-term fat loss comes from improving our basic biological functions rather than fighting against them. We improve them by increasing the quality of calories we eat and the quality of exercises we do.
- Temporary weight loss comes from ignoring our clog while fiddling with the quantity of calories we take in and exercise off. Temporary weight

loss comes from making our body think it is starving. This approach causes us to slow down, hold on to body fat, burn muscle, and gain back more body fat than we lost.

- Studies show that the calorie myths—counting calories, believing that a calorie is a calorie, saying that calories are all that matter, and the rest—fail because they ignore the set-point, calorie quality, and our hormonal clog. The calorie myths ignore all the factors controlling long-term health and fat loss. That is why studies show they fail more than 95 percent of the time.

- By focusing on calorie quality, we eat as much SANE—high-Satiety, low-Aggression, high-Nutrition, and low-Efficiency—food as possible, and sit back while our body takes care of itself. Our hormones get healed, our clog clears, our set-point drops, and we burn body fat all day, automatically.

- Eating SANE food is simple. We eat natural whole foods packed with water, fiber, protein, and essential fats. We eat the way our ancestors ate for 99.8 percent of our history. We eat the way people ate before obesity and all its related diseases became a problem.

- Sadly, our government promotes disproved, imbalanced, and unnatural dietary guidelines that encourage the inSANE eating that causes obesity, diabetes, and heart disease.

- Big food, fitness, and pharmaceutical corporations pile on the inSANE "food" and spread misinformation because the worse we do, the better they do.

- We do not burn more body fat by exercising more. We burn more body fat by unclogging. We unclog by working more muscle fibers and triggering clog-clearing hormones. This type of smarter exercise is performed by moving forcefully, briefly, infrequently, and safely. Exercise helps us burn body fat forever when we do less of it—smarter.

- Eating less and exercising more to manually balance calories is complex and counterproductive. Eating more and exercising less—but smarter—to enable our body to balance calories for us makes slim simple.

- Eating more SANE food provides the unique combination of more nutrients, more satisfaction, and more clog clearing, while preventing us from overeating. Add in smarter exercise and we stimulate our clog-clearing hormones. More nutrients plus less overeating and less clogging quickly convince our body to lower our set-point and burn body fat for us automatically. Since we will heal our mind along with our body while eating *more* and exercising *less* than ever, we can easily keep this up long term.

The science is simple. The lifestyle is easy. The results are amazing. Here's to a lifetime of fighting fat with facts instead of getting frustrated by fat-loss fiction.

Afterword: Spread the Word
(and Get Bonus Content!)

We cannot solve problems by using the same kind of thinking we used when we created them.

—Albert Einstein

In the past, the "truth" about our diet and fitness has been determined by a number of factors, including market forces. This no longer has to be the case. The truth can be determined by science. You and I simply need to get the word out. If every one of us spends a few seconds sharing this scientific news, we can create a healthier and happier world.

—Jonathan Bailor

Free Recipes, Meal Plans, Exercise Videos, How-To Videos, eBooks, and More
Get delicious recipes, at-home exercise videos, simple meal plans, and personalized support at www.SANESolution.com.

New FAQs for the Updated Edition

Since the initial publication of *The Calorie Myth,* readers have consistently asked what we should track if not calories, how they can get started immediately, how SANE eating differs from traditional calorie-counting programs, and how this all got started. Answers and action steps for all of these questions are provided here, and please visit www.SANESolution.com for additional updates, free bonuses, and to get your free personalized program today.

QUESTION 1: I FIND TRACKING WHAT I EAT HELPFUL. SHOULD I STOP?

Tracking what you eat has been shown to help with long-term fat loss and health. The issue is not with keeping tabs on what you are eating. The issue is with evaluating your success using obsolete measures such as calories.

When you use conventional calorie-counting tools, you are forced to ignore everything about food except the quantity of energy those foods provide. According to these obsolete tools, you would be better off eating 21 teaspoons of sugar than eating an avocado, as the 21 teaspoons of sugar have fewer calories. This is insane. Why not track using a modern measurement that considers all aspects of food that impact your weight and health? Great idea, but easier said than done, as no such system existed when this book was initially published.

That has all changed now. There is a SANE alternative to calories. Just like you can see your calorie count for a meal over time and set calorie goals, you can now see the SANEity of your meals over time, and how you are doing relative to your goals. Instead of spending a lot of time tracking the quantity of energy you are putting into your body and ignoring everything else, you can spend a little time tracking both the quantity and quality of what you are eating. You can access this new patent-pending technology and see, score, and share your SANEity using your free app and online program at www.SANE Solution.com. I hope it's helpful!

QUESTION 2: WHAT CAN I START DOING TODAY TO LOSE WEIGHT AND FEEL BETTER?

These are the top three things you can start doing right now to heal your body and your mind:

1. ENJOY DELICIOUS FOOD: Your dinner table is for savoring and smiles, not self-criticism and calorie math. Eating should be a source of joy, not shame. Eat *more* whole foods to burn more body fat.
2. HEAL YOUR BODY AND MIND: Obesity isn't a character flaw. It is a disease like diabetes. Don't try to starve your body by engaging with incorrect information. Instead, start leveraging whole foods to heal yourself and live better.
3. SIMPLIFY AND CONNECT: Healthy cannot be complex. We were slimmer before we started counting calories. Say goodbye to complex calorie counting and hello to real, delicious food. If tracking what you are eating is helpful, simply take photos of your meals and share the photos on your social networks. This will help you focus on food quality instead of calorie quantity, and will also help you stay motivated and accountable by involving your friends. You can do this simply and see the SANEity of your meals with your free SANE app at www.SANESolution.com.

QUESTION 3: HOW IS THIS PROGRAM DIFFERENT FROM OTHER WEIGHT-LOSS PROGRAMS?

The SANE approach to weight loss is an abundance-based approach rooted in modern science. Conventional programs offer traditional calorie- and willpower-based approaches that simply don't work, and often leave you feeling like you never get enough to eat. The last fifty years have provided radical scientific and technological advancements in every area of our lives. Finding new ways to enjoyably burn fat and boost health is no exception.

Going SANE is all about leveraging modern science and technology to achieve your wellness goals based on the proven philosophy that:

- Chronic fat gain, diabetes, and related diseases are caused by a breakdown of your brain, hormones, and gut.
- This breakdown is caused by eating processed products and low-quality foods that provide too much of the things you don't need (such as sugar, MSG, and trans fat), and too little of the things you do need (including vitamins, minerals, and essential proteins and fats).
- Modern psychology and biology prove that by eating an abundance of delicious and nutritious whole foods via a fun, simple, and social program, you can burn fat and boost health simply and sustainably.

Conventional calories-in-calories-out programs are rooted in the fifty-year-old theory that weight gain is caused by a lack of willpower. Despite the fact that studies show that overweight people eat no more than lean people, these conventional programs use negative reinforcement approaches, such as starvation dieting and public weigh-ins, all based on the belief that weight gain is a character flaw and can be addressed by shaming people. They generally lead to short-term weight loss followed by long-term fat gain, crippling psychological issues, and eating disorders.

Conventional Calorie-Counting Programs	Your SANE Solution
Eating is portrayed as something to be avoided.	Eating is celebrated.
You use fifty-year-old technology and biology to make wellness decisions.	You leverage modern technology and biology to eat more high-quality SANE food.
You use willpower to reduce the number of calories you eat—regardless of their source—never addressing the biological causes of obesity.	You use your phone to snap and share food photos to increase the quality/SANEity of food you eat, and heal the biological causes of obesity and diabetes.
You will temporarily lose weight, but over 95% of people will yo-yo diet.	You will sustainably burn fat, speed up your metabolism, avoid hunger, increase energy levels, and avoid overeating.
You will put less water in your still "clogged" metabolic sink.	You will "unclog" your metabolic sink.

QUESTION 4: HOW DID THIS GET STARTED?

Once upon a time there was a skinny, geeky little boy who wanted to be Superman. OK, that kid was me. Growing up, I always idolized my big brother, a strong football player. Every night I sat at the dinner table with him and my super-brainy professor parents, dreaming of the day that I would be as tall and strong as my brother. But as birthdays came and went, the opposite happened—I grew taller and lankier, not bigger and stronger.

So I did what any professors' kid would do: I studied, devouring health and fitness magazines and books, listening to big, strong men like my brother talk about how to get big and strong. I thought I had finally discovered the secret to becoming Superman, so when I went to college, I decided to put some of this hard-earned knowledge to work by trying to help other people change their bodies as a personal trainer. Every day I ate more calories, trying to gain weight—to become bigger. And every day I would ask my clients to eat less, so they could lose weight—to become smaller.

I ate up to 6,000 calories a day and did no cardiovascular exercise. And yet I didn't gain an ounce. Meanwhile, my clients would eat 1,600 calories and exercise for half an hour each day. And they couldn't lose a pound. So I cut them down to 1,400 calories and increased their workouts to an hour a day. Then down to 1,200 calories and hour-and-a-half workouts every day. And their weight still didn't budge.

My clients felt more and more miserable—achy, angry, and even depressed. I did too. I couldn't help myself, and I couldn't help them. In private moments of frustration, I admit I blamed my clients. "If they could just eat less, they would lose weight—what's their problem?" I thought. "They just need to try harder!"

One day, while I drank a shot of calorie-packed olive oil, it suddenly occurred to me: What if some big, strong man out there was thinking the exact same thing about *me*? "If that skinny, geeky kid could just eat more, he would gain weight—what's his problem? He just needs to try harder." In that moment, I realized that even though all I'd ever wanted to do was help people feel healthier and better about themselves, what I was doing was making everyone—including myself—sicker and sadder. I was determined to make things right.

So I asked my parents for advice. I told them about the countless hours I'd spent reading and studying and applying what I'd learned—and the results I wasn't seeing. And they said, "You and your clients are not suffering from an effort problem. You're all trying really hard. What you have is an information problem. Consider the source."

I threw away everything I thought I knew and started fresh, beginning a new journey that took me deep into the foreign and little-traveled lands of jargon-packed scientific studies and mind-bending academic journal articles. In the process, I discovered that everything I'd ever been taught as a trainer was disproven in the scientific literature. Every single thing I thought I knew about fitness and weight loss was wrong.

As I learned more, I was no longer interested in fighting against the body; I wanted to learn how to *transform* the body. I wanted to learn how to improve the system itself, rather than use barbaric supplementation or starvation to torture a system that wasn't working correctly in the first place.

Ten years, 10,000 pages of research, 1,300 scientific studies, and countless conversations with scientists later, I emerged from my research journey reborn. For the first time, I realized a stark truth: I would never become Superman. My genes simply wouldn't allow it. But I also realized a truth that freed me and changed my life forever: while I might never become Superman, through modern eating and exercise science, I could become the very best version of the person I was born to be.

Once I realized how the body really works, I couldn't wait to share the information with the world. I recommitted my life to helping people achieve their weight-loss goals with data and facts, rather than hurting them with fairy tales of starvation dieting and binge eating. The bottom line is: you can transform your body. You can enjoy an astounding level of vibrancy, love, and satisfaction in your life. You can eat more, not less—and you will get leaner and healthier in the process. You don't have to suffer. You just need the correct information.

You just need to go SANE—and then you will become super, too. And you and your body will truly live happily ever after.

Acknowledgments

This book is the result of more than twelve years of collaboration with hundreds of brilliant and inspiring researchers. To everyone who helped bring this science to the surface: I cannot thank you enough for your time, insight, and support. Together we will make the world a healthier and happier place.

To my agent, Linda Konner: you have exceeded my wildest expectations. Thank you for helping make my dreams come true. Thank you to the tremendous team at HarperCollins and beyond for facilitating this once-in-a-lifetime opportunity. To my executive editor, Julie Will, your passion and commitment to this project were obvious and inspiring from day one. Thank you for your unwavering support and trust and for the immeasurable value you added to this project. You exceeded expectations every step of the way. To Mariska van Aalst: what you do with words is nothing short of magical. Thank you for waving your wondrous wordsmithing wand my way. To marketing director Katie O'Callaghan and my publicist, Kate D'Esmond: modern nutrition and exercise science is only as helpful as it is available to the public. Thank you for the passion and creativity you bring to making this lifesaving research accessible to everyone.

Thank you to the most incredible person I have ever met in my life. My best friend, my partner, my everything, my wife, Angela. Every day I'm met with wonderment as to how I am so lucky to spend my life and my forever with such an angelic being. This book and the broader dream it reflects would not exist were it not for your remarkable support and collaboration.

Thank you to Scott, Zeyad, Mike, Kevin, Cameron, and Branden; my delightful sister, Patty; my loving in-laws, Terry and Carolyn; and my big brother and best man, Tim. You are such treasures. Thank you for being who you are, and thank you for meaning so much to me.

Thank you to my dazzling podcast cohost and SANE chef Carrie Brown. You bring so much joy on so many levels to so many people. Thank you for being the gem that you are.

Thank you to my enlightened mentor and business partner, Joshua Pokempner. You are an angel in every sense of the word. Thank you for giving so much of yourself to such a noble mission.

Thank you to my amazing support group moderator, brilliant content provider, and medical adviser Dr. Catherine W. Britell. Thank you for your consistent and dependable time, insight, and caring.

Thank you to Dr. JoAnn E. Manson, Dr. Theodoros Kelesidis, and Dr. William Davis for your life-changing research and collaboration. And to Tom Naughton, Lisa Johnson, Jimmy Moore, Sean Croxton, Mark Sisson, Lynn Colwell, Corey Colwell-Lipson, Jade Teta, Able James, Ben Greenfield, JJ Virgin, Laura Dolson, Dave Asprey, Pilar Gerasimo, A. J. Jacobs, Casey Carey, John Carey, Brian Johnson, David Moldawer, Michael Karsh, Jeska Dzwigalski, Elizabeth Madariaga, Dr. Josh Axe, Nicholas Robinson, Dr. Mark Hyman, Anne McLaughlin, Dr. Christiane Northrup, Diane Grover, Dr. Daniel G. Amen, Dr. Michael Moreno, Dr. John Berardi, Dr. Lauren Streicher, Darya Rose, Melissa Hartwig, Dr. David L. Katz, Dr. Barry Sears, Robert Goodman, Diane Sanfilippo, Adam Bornstein, Dietitian Cassie, Steve Wright, Becca Borawski, Dr. Sara Gottfried, Kate Ferguson, Lawren Pulse, Dr. Stephan Guyenet, Mareya Ibrahim, Mira and Jayson Calton, Nell Stephenson, Richard Nikoley, Dr. Ray Hinish, Monica Reinagel, Dr. Fred Pescatore, Dr. Andreas Eenfeldt, and the teams at the *Huffington Post,* en*theos, Quest Nutrition, BeWell Radio, and creativeLIVE, for your insightful work, for your dedication to making "healthy" healthy again, for helping me find my way in the world of social media, and for supporting me every step of the way.

Thank you to the amazing team behind our nonprofit efforts at Blare Media and beyond: Mike Rich, Justin McAleece, Johnny Soto, Jason Wada, and Jennifer Barnett. Your generosity and brilliance have improved the lives of so many so deeply.

Thank you to the editors of the first edition of this book: John Paine, Hillel Black, Mary Rose Bailor, and Robert Bailor. I consider you magicians more than editors. Your brilliance is exceeded only by your kindness.

Thank you to the amazing teams at DigiPowers Inc., Krupp Kommunications Inc., and Sarah Wilson Business Communications. Rolf Kaiser, Jacob Waldman, Corey McCraw, Brian Toomey, Aaron Mandelbaum, Ken Reid, Alex Borsody, Brian Bason, Julia Miller, Jim Miller, Heidi Krupp, Sarah Wilson, and Mark Fortier: your creativity and diligence have enabled us to make "healthy" healthy again at a whole new level.

Thank you to my marvelous Microsoft management team: Tristan Davis, Scott Stiles, Jeanne Sheldon, Michelle Tatom, Stacey Law, Samara Donald, and Jessica Zahn for enabling me to live out my dreams of simplifying and applying technology and biology for the betterment of humanity. Your ongoing support for this science is nothing short of amazing.

Thank you to Robert, Jay, Jennifer, Cristina, Char, Jim, and Carrie for sharing your SANE success stories and for setting such an inspirational example.

Thank you to Sheri Ackerman, John Coss, Caitlin Ashley-Rollman, LeAnne

Marshall, Angela Streiff, Robby Reining, Robert Bailor, Angela Bailor, Melinda Knight, Alan Hukle, Craig Stephans, Cherie Hill, Julie Spiegel, Bill Cashell, Lydia Allen, Angie Boyter, John Roberto, Tara Hopwood, Michael David McGuire, and Andrew Warner for your substantial and insightful feedback. I hope this text lives up to your inspiring expectations.

Finally, thank you to every member of the SANE communities worldwide. The support you have shown from day one has consistently caused me to get teary eyed. You have the courage to go SANE and exercise smarter. You have taken the road less traveled and it will make all the difference.

Appendix A:
To Do before Exercising Smarter

BY CATHERINE W. BRITELL, MD

Starting a new exercise program is exciting. You can look forward to getting stronger, having more energy, and looking better. However, if you have some uncertainty about your cardiovascular health, you may have well-founded concerns about whether it's safe to begin a new exercise program.

If you have had symptoms such as chest pain or irregular heart rhythm, or had a heart attack or a coronary artery stent or bypass, you must consult with your doctor before trying any new vigorous exercises. In addition, consulting with your physician is especially important if you:

- Are over forty
- Have diabetes
- Smoke
- Have high blood pressure (above 140 systolic and/or 90 diastolic)
- Have high LDL cholesterol and triglycerides and low HDL cholesterol
- Have a waist circumference greater than 32 inches in women and 37 inches in men
- Are sedentary

The good news is that both high-intensity interval training and eccentric strengthening have been shown to be excellent ways for individuals with cardiac problems to become healthier and stronger, if started and monitored carefully in a supervised program of cardiac rehabilitation.

The bottom line: see your doctor before starting any kind of new exercise program, and bring along a concise outline of the exercises you plan to do. If you have cardiovascular risk factors, a cardiology consultation and possible cardiac stress testing are the best way to ensure your getting into your new exercise program safely. If you have cardiac abnormalities, high-intensity interval training and eccentric strengthening may be very effective, provided they are done with appropriate cardiac monitoring on recommendation of your cardiologist.

Appendix B:
Products That Make Going
SANE More Convenient

Every day we see some new "must have" pill or powder promising to transform our health. Every day we need to remind ourselves that none of these products could possibly be required to avoid obesity, diabetes, and heart disease. None of us are overweight or sick owing to a pill or powder deficiency. How could we be? These products didn't exist until recently and neither did rampant obesity, diabetes, and heart disease. Obesity and disease are caused by a deficiency of SANE foods and a surplus of inSANE edible products. Everything essential for human health is found within SANE whole foods—to the extent that if we eat more of them we will avoid obesity and disease without trying.

That said, there are some products that may make staying SANE and getting eccentric easier. The brands that I use and trust can be found on The Smarter Science of Slim website. Note that I am not receiving any compensation from anyone for these recommendations. None of them are required. They simply save some people time and money in the long term.

MEMBERSHIP AT A BULK WHOLESALE STORE: With the cash-back "executive" memberships many of these stores offer, you can end up getting paid to become a member. My wife and I really like Costco.

HIGH-QUALITY BLENDER: If you want to make smoothies, a good blender costs between $300 and $400. If you blend frequently, cheap blenders cost you more over the long run because they have to be replaced frequently.

You will also find that high-quality blenders are significantly better at making tasty smoothies. Cheap blenders break food into small chunks, and it is no fun drinking grainy, chunky smoothies. High-quality blenders create smooth and delightful smoothies. For example, if you put spinach into a $100 blender, you will get bits of spinach. However, if you put spinach into a $350 blender, you will get smooth spinach juice. Or consider whole flaxseed. Cheap blenders mix this up and leave you with whole seeds. High-quality blenders liquefy it. If you had a grainy, chunky, and overall bad experience with blending in the past, blame the blender and give smoothies another shot with a better blender.

I use a refurbished Vitamix blender, which costs a little under $350. There are other great ones out there. I chose the Vitamix because it has an impressive seven-year warranty and comes with a large jar—to blend a lot at once—and a handy plunger, to push food down in the blender without splattering it all over the place. If your time is scarce, I think a $350 blender is worth the investment. If it lasts you seven years—which it will if it has a seven-year warranty—that is $50 a year.

BULK UNSWEETENED AND UNDUTCHED COCOA/CACAO: If you like chocolate, buying unsweetened cocoa/cacao in bulk is a great cost saver. Unlike chocolate, pure cocoa/cacao is one of the most SANE foods in the world.

INDOOR GRILL: A must-have for easy meat and seafood preparation. George Foreman's is the most common. There are other great ones. My only recommendation is to get one where you can detach the grilling "plates" for easy washing.

SHAKER BOTTLES: These are helpful for enjoying green smoothies on the go.

PULL-UP BAR: These cost less than $50, can be installed in any doorway, and make at-home eccentric back exercises simple.

LIFTING GLOVES AND STRAPS: These protect your hands and wrists while enabling you to grip resistance more securely when exercising eccentrically.

HEAVY RESISTANCE BANDS: These are inexpensive, portable, and versatile ways to add resistance to at-home eccentric exercise.

ADJUSTABLE WEIGHT VEST: This is another way to add resistance to at-home eccentric exercises.

SUGAR-FREE POWDERED "SUPER FOODS": These offer a convenient but horrible-tasting way to get nonstarchy vegetables and low-fructose fruits when whole-food options aren't available.

LOW-SUGAR PROTEIN BARS: These should contain at least five times more protein than sugar. Also, the fewer ingredients, the better the bar. Note that the vast majority of bars out there contain more sugar than anything else and should be avoided.

CASEIN OR WHEY PROTEIN POWDER: Many supplement companies advertise that their whey protein is best. Do not believe the hype. Just make sure your protein powder does not contain a bunch of extra ingredients. Any product with more than two grams of sugar per twenty-five grams of protein is low-quality and should be avoided.

When choosing flavors, think about how you are going to eat the protein. If you plan to blend it with fruits and vegetables, then I recommend vanilla, strawberry, or some other fruit flavor. Other flavors are risky with low-fructose fruits and nonstarchy vegetables. If you plan on mixing the protein with only water, ice, and whole-food fats, get whatever flavor sounds appealing to you.

If you plan to use the powder before and after workouts, go with whey given its rapid rate of digestion. Otherwise, stick with casein, as it is the less Aggressive of the two.

If you prefer to avoid dairy, and as long as you are not using the powder to add flavor, powdered egg whites can also be used given their casein- and whey-like rich and complete amino acid profile.

MANDOLINE: This will save you a lot of time chopping nonstarchy vegetables.

SLICING GLOVES: These will save your fingers while you are chopping nonstarchy vegetables.

STAND-ALONE FREEZER: If many people in your house are going SANE, a stand-alone freezer is helpful. All this freezer space allows you to buy nonstarchy vegetables, meats, seafood, and fruits in bulk, and saves you money and time.

Appendix C:
Further Reading

The resources listed here reflect a wide array of lifestyles that have helped millions of people live better. As you enjoy the diversity of eating and exercise strategies found in this list, please keep the proven science and simple principles we've covered in mind. Most important, remember that the worldwide rate of obesity has more than doubled since 1980, the rate of diabetes and prediabetes has increased 100,000 percent in one century, and more than 40 million children under the age of five are overweight. Nobody working to help others eat nutrient-dense food instead of manufactured edible products is our adversary. We're here to be healthy and to enjoy our lives, not to argue over ideology. Biology isn't a matter of opinion anyway.

Let's focus our time on health, happiness, helping others, and celebrating similarities rather than demonizing differences. *Together* we can turn the tide against the worst health crisis the modern world has ever seen. And we must. It is a matter of life and death.

Note: Since websites change but books don't, listed below are the names of authors, bloggers, broadcasters, and others who have influenced me. To enjoy their most recent work, type any of the names, surrounded by quotation marks, into your favorite search engine.

A. J. Jacobs
Chef AJ
Abel James
Adam Bornstein
Adam Kosloff
Aglaée Jacob
Alexandra Jamieson
Amy Mac
Andrea Beaman
Andrew S. Rockoff
Aran Goyoaga

Arsy Vartanian
Ashley Borden
Ashley Koff
Barton Seaver
Becca Borawski
Ben Coomber
Ben Greenfield
Brandi Koskie
Brenda Wollenberg
Brett Klika
Bridgit Danner

Brierley Wright
Carol Salva
Carole Carson
Caryn Hartglass
Caryn Talty
Cate Ritter
Catherine Holecko
Charlie Hoehn
Christa Orecchio
Christie Johnson
Christine Biswabic

Corey Colwell-Lipson

Cynthia Pasquella

Dan Ariely

Dan Millman

Daphne Oz

Dave Asprey

David Barr

Debra-Lynn B. Hook

Dee McCaffrey

Denise Mestanza-Taylor

Diane Sanfilippo

Dick Bolles

Dietitian Cassie

Donna Gates

Doug Cook

Dr. Alice D. Domar

Dr. Andreas Eenfeldt

Dr. Barbara Natterson-
  Horowitz

Dr. Barry Sears

Dr. Brad Blanton

Dr. Carol S. Dweck

Dr. Christiane Northrup

Dr. Colin Champ

Dr. Daniel Amen

Dr. Daniel Kalish

Dr. Darya Rose

Dr. David L. Katz

Dr. Drew Ramsey

Dr. Dwight Lundell

Dr. Edmund J. Bourne

Dr. Fred Pescatore

Dr. George Pratt

Dr. Holly Lucille

Dr. Jacob Teitelbaum

Dr. Jade Teta

Dr. Jay Wortman

Dr. Jeffry N. Gerber

Dr. Jeffry S. Life

Dr. Jim Nicolai

Dr. Joel Furhman

Dr. John Berardi

Dr. John Gottman

Dr. John J. Ratey

Dr. Jonny Bowden

Dr. Kelly Austin

Dr. Kelly Starrett

Dr. Larry Dossey

Dr. Lauren F. Streicher

Dr. Lori L. Shemek

Dr. Mao Shing Ni

Dr. Mark Hyman

Dr. Joseph M. Mercola

Dr. Michael Terman

Dr. Mike Moreno

Dr. Mike Young

Dr. Natasha Turner

Dr. Neal Barnard

Dr. Nicole M. Avena

Dr. Nina Savelle-Rocklin

Dr. Peter Attia

Dr. Rallie McAllister

Dr. Ray Hinish

Dr. Richard Johnson

Dr. Rick Henriksen

Dr. Robert J. Davis

Dr. Ron Rosedale

Dr. Sara Gottfried

Dr. Sarah Ballantyne

Dr. Srdjan Ostric

Dr. Stephan Guyenet

Dr. T. Colin Campbell

Dr. Terri Orbuch

Dr. Terry Wahls

Dr. Tom O'Bryan

Dr. Vera Ingrid Tarman

Dr. Walter Willett

Dr. Wayne Westcott

Dr. Will Tuttle

Dr. William Davis

Elise Ballard

Elliott Hulse

Eric Cressey

Esther Blum

Esther Horn

FitBuff Brandon

Frances Largeman-Roth

Gary Noreen

Gary Taubes

George Bryant

Georgina Ryan

Ginger Vieira

Gretchen Rubin

Gunnar Peterson

Guy Kawasaki

Howard Jacobson

Jack Canfield

Jackie Eberstein

Jay Jacobs

Jayson and Mira Calton

Jennifer Bright Reich

Jennifer Knye

Jennipher Walters

Jeremy Hendon

Jill Escher

Jimmy Moore

JJ Virgin

Joe and Terry Graedon

Joel Harper

John Kiefer

John Little

Jonathan Haidt

Joy Houston

Joyce Richey

Julia Cameron

Justin Smith

Karen Asp

Kate Ferguson

Kate Finley

Kathryn Budig

Kathy Freston

Kathy Smart

Katy Bowman

Keri Gans
Kevin Cann
Kevin Carroll Katalyst
Kimberly Hartke
Kris Gunnars
Krista Scott-Dixon
Laura Dolson
Lawren Pulse
Lesley Alderman
Lierre Keith
Linda Melone
Lindsay Vastola
Lisa Cain
Lisa Johnson
Lisa Lillien
Liz Weiss and Janice
   Newell Bissex
Liz Wolfe
Lynda Scott
Lyn-Genet Recitas
Lynn Colwell
Mareya Ibrahim
Mark Sisson
Mark Spurbeck
Maya Nahra
Meghann Douglas
Melissa Hartwig
Melissa Joulwan

Michael Boyle
Michelle Curtis Norris
Michele Simon
Michelle Fagone
Mike Reinold
Monica Reinagel
Neely Quinn
Nell Stephenson
Nia Shanks
Nick Evans
Nicki Anderson
Nickie Cochran
Nina Planck
Nora Gedgaudas
Paul Jaminet
Peggy Kotsopoulos
Perry Romanowski
Prof. Gary L. Wenk
Prof. Hamilton M. Stapell
Prof. Timothy Noakes
Rachel Cosgrove
Ray Audette
Rebecca Rider
Reed Davis
Reinhard Engels
Richard Nikoley
Robert Greene
Rolf Dobelli

Rory Freedman
Sam Feltham
Sam Feltham
Sean Croxton
Sean Hyson
Shawn Stevenson
Shirley Braden
Stacy Toth
Stanley Fishman
Steve Kamb
Steve Wright and Jordan
   Reasoner
Stuart McRobert
Suzane Bowen
Tal Ben-Shahar
Tana Amen
Tara Grant
Ted Spiker
Thea H. Singer
Timothy Caulfield
Tom Naughton
Tony Gaskins
Tony Gentilcore
Tricia Greaves Nelson
Troy Casey
Vinnie Tortorich
Wayne Parcelle
William J. Broad

Notes

This book is the simplification and application of more than twelve hundred academic studies. The complete list of supporting scientific literature can be found broken down into the following six subjects on TheCalorieMythBook .com:

- Set-Point: Homeostatic Regulation of Body Weight
- A Calorie Is Not a Calorie: SANE Calories
- Why Hormones Matter: The Moderation Myth
- Calorie Counting Is Unnecessary and Ineffective
- SANE Eating: Eating More—Smarter
- Smarter Exercise: Exercising Less—Smarter

The sources for key studies and direct quotations in the text are provided below.

1. Jensen, AR. "How Much Can We Boost IQ and Scholastic Achievement?" *Harvard Educ Rev* 39 (1969): 1–123.
2. Belluck, Pam. "Children's Life Expectancy Being Cut Short by Obesity." *The New York Times*, June 3, 2012, http://www.nytimes.com/2005/03/17/health/17obese.html.
3. Wooley, SC, and DM Garner. "Dietary Treatments for Obesity Are Ineffective." *BMJ* 309(6955) (1994): 655–56; PubMed PMID: 8086992; PubMed Central PMCID: PMC2541482.
4. Stunkard, A, and M McClaren-Hume. "The Results of Treatment for Obesity: A Review of the Literature and a Report of a Series." *Archives of Internal Medicine* 103(I) (1959): 79–85.
5. Friedman, JM. "Modern Science versus the Stigma of Obesity." *Nat Med* 10(6) (2004): 563–69; review; PubMed PMID: 15170194.
6. Ibid.
7. Wisse, BE, and MW Schwartz. "Does Hypothalamic Inflammation Cause Obesity?" *Cell Metab* 10(4) (2009): 241–42; PubMed PMID: 19808014.
8. Miller, WC, AK Lindeman, J Wallace, and M Niederpruem. "Diet Compo-

sition, Energy Intake, and Exercise in Relation to Body Fat in Men and Women." *Am J Clin Nutr* 52(3) (1990): 426–30; PubMed PMID: 2393005.

9. Friedman. "Modern Science versus the Stigma of Obesity."

10. Weigle, DS. "Human Obesity: Exploding the Myths." *West J Med* 153(4) (1990): 421–28; review; PubMed PMID: 2244378; PubMed Central PMCID: PMC1002573.

11. Roberts, Paul. *The End of Food*. Boston: Houghton Mifflin, 2008.

12. Weigle, DS. "Appetite and the Regulation of Body Composition." *FASEB J* 8(3) (1994): 302–10; review; PubMed PMID: 8143936.

13. Sumithran, P, LA Prendergast, E Delbridge, K Purcell, A Shulkes, A Kriketos, J Proietto. "Long-Term Persistence of Hormonal Adaptations to Weight Loss." *N Engl J Med* 365(17) (2011): 1597–604; doi: 10.1056/NEJMoa 1105816; PubMed PMID: 22029981.

14. Ibid.

15. Keesey, RE, and MD Hirvonen. "Body Weight Set-Points: Determination and Adjustment." *J Nutr* 127(9) (1997): 1875S–83S; review; PubMed PMID: 9278574.

16. Rolls, BJ, EA Rowe, and RC Turner. "Persistent Obesity in Rats Following a Period of Consumption of a Mixed, High Energy Diet." *J Physiol* 298 (1980): 415–27; PubMed PMID: 6987379; PubMed Central PMCID: PMC1279126.

17. Ibid.

18. Everard, A, V Lazarevic, M Derrien, M Girard, GG Muccioli, AM Neyrinck, S Possemiers, A Van Holle, P François, WM de Vos, NM Delzenne, J Schrenzel, and PD Cani. "Responses of Gut Microbiota and Glucose and Lipid Metabolism to Prebiotics in Genetic Obese and Diet-Induced Leptin-Resistant Mice." *Diabetes* 60(11) (2011): 2775–86; doi: 10.2337/db11–0227; Epub September 20, 2011; erratum in *Diabetes* 60(12) (2011): 3307, Muccioli, Giulio M (corrected to Muccioli, Giulio G); PubMed PMID: 21933985; PubMed Central PMCID: PMC3198091.

19. Morrison, CD, and H-R Berthoud. "Neurobiology of Nutrition and Obesity." *Nutr Rev* 65(12 pt 1) (2007): 517–34; review; PubMed PMID: 18236691.

20. Interview with Stephan Guyenet, June 4, 2013; his blog is at http://www .blogger.com/profile/09218114625524777250.

21. A sampling of supporting research includes the following studies: Westman, EC, WS Yancy Jr, MD Haub, and JS Volek, "Insulin Resistance from a Low-Carbohydrate, High Fat Diet Perspective." *Metabolic Syndrome and Related Disorders* 3 (2005): 3–7; Boden, G, K Sargrad, C Homko, M Mozzoli, and TP Stein, "Effect of a Low-Carbohydrate Diet on Appetite, Blood Glucose Levels, and Insulin Resistance in Obese Patients with Type 2 Diabetes." *Ann Intern Med* 142(6) (2005): 403–11; Nielsen, JV, and EA Jöns-

son, "Low-Carbohydrate Diet in Type 2 Diabetes: Stable Improvement of Bodyweight and Glycaemic Control during 22 Months Follow-Up." *Nutr Metab* (Lond) 3(1) (2006): 22; Eaton, SB, L Cordain, and PB Sparling, "Evolution, Body Composition, Insulin Receptor Competition, and Insulin Resistance." *Prev Med* 49(4) (2009): 283–85, Epub August 15, 2009, PubMed PMID: 19686772; Craig, BW, J Everhart, and R Brown, "The Influence of High-Resistance Training on Glucose Tolerance in Young and Elderly Subjects." *Mech Ageing Dev* 49(2) (1989): 147–57, review, PubMed PMID: 2677535; Miller, WJ, WM Sherman, and JL Ivy, "Effect of Strength Training on Glucose Tolerance and Post-Glucose Insulin Response." *Med Sci Sports Exerc* 16(6) (1984): 539–43, PubMed PMID: 6392812.

22. Everard et al. "Responses of Gut Microbiota."

23. Everard, A, C Belzer, L Geurts, JP Ouwerkerk, C Druart, LB Bindels, Y Guiot, M Derrien, GG Muccioli, NM Delzenne, WM de Vos, PD Cani. "Cross-Talk between Akkermansia Muciniphila and Intestinal Epithelium Controls Diet-Induced Obesity." *Proc Natl Acad Sci U S A* 110(22) (2013): 9066–71; doi: 10.1073/pnas.1219451110; Epub May 13, 2013; PubMed PMID: 23671105.

24. Peck, JW. "Rats Defend Different Body Weights Depending on Palatability and Accessibility of Their Food." *J Comp Physiol Psychol* 92(3) (1978): 555–70; PubMed PMID: 98538.

25. Rothwell, NJ, and MJ Stock. "Energy Expenditure of 'Cafeteria'-Fed Rats Determined from Measurements of Energy Balance and Indirect Calorimetry." *J Physiol* 328 (1982): 371–77; PubMed PMID: 7131317; PubMed Central PMCID: PMC1225664.

26. Howard, BV, JE Manson, ML Stefanick, SA Beresford, G Frank, B Jones, RJ Rodabough, L Snetselaar, C Thomson, L Tinker, M Vitolins, and R Prentice. "Low-Fat Dietary Pattern and Weight Change over 7 Years: The Women's Health Initiative Dietary Modification Trial." *JAMA* 295(1) (2006): 39–49; PubMed PMID: 16391215.

27. Thorpe, GL. "Treating Overweight Patients." *J Am Med Assoc* 165(11) (1957): 1361–65; PubMed PMID: 13475044.

28. Feinman, RD, and EJ Fine. "'A Calorie Is a Calorie' Violates the Second Law of Thermodynamics." *Nutr J* 3 (July 28, 2004): 9; PubMed PMID: 15282028; PubMed Central PMCID: PMC506782.

29. Young, EA, MM Harris, TL Cantu, JJ Ghidoni, and R Crawley. "Hepatic Response to a Very-Low-Energy Diet and Refeeding in Rats." *Am J Clin Nutr* 57(6) (1993): 857–62; PubMed PMID: 8503353.

30. Leibel, RL, and J Hirsch. "Diminished Energy Requirements in Reduced-Obese Patients." *Metabolism* 33(2) (1984): 164–70; PubMed PMID: 6694559.

31. Keesey, RE, and TL Powley. "The Regulation of Body Weight." *Annu Rev Psychol* 37 (1986): 109–33; PubMed PMID: 3963779.

32. Garrow, JS. "The Safety of Dieting." *Proc Nutr Soc* 50(2) (1991): 493–99; review; PubMed PMID: 1749815.

33. Garner, DM, and SC Wooley. "Confronting the Failure of Behavioral and Dietary Treatments for Obesity." *Clin Psychol Rev* 11 (1991): 729–80; doi: 10.1016/0272-7358(91)90128-H.

34. Blackburn, GL, GT Wilson, BS Kanders, LJ Stein, PT Lavin, J Adler, and KD Brownell. "Weight Cycling: The Experience of Human Dieters." *Am J Clin Nutr* 49(5 Suppl) (1989): 1105–1109; PubMed PMID: 2718940.

35. McCullough, ML, D Feskanich, MJ Stampfer, BA Rosner, FB Hu, DJ Hunter, JN Variyam, GA Colditz, and WC Willett. "Adherence to the *Dietary Guidelines for Americans* and Risk of Major Chronic Disease in Women." *Am J Clin Nutr* 72(5) (2000): 1214–22; PubMed PMID: 11063452.

36. Mann, T, AJ Tomiyama, E Westling, AM Lew, B Samuels, and J Chatman. "Medicare's Search for Effective Obesity Treatments: Diets Are Not the Answer." *Am Psychol* 62(3) (2007): 220–33; review; PubMed PMID: 17469900.

37. Weigle, DS. "Human Obesity: Exploding the Myths." *West J Med* 153(4) (1990): 421–28; review; PubMed PMID: 2244378; PubMed Central PMCID: PMC1002573.

38. Volek, J, M Sharman, A Gómez, D Judelson, M Rubin, G Watson, B Sokmen, R Silvestre, D French, and W Kraemer. "Comparison of Energy-Restricted Very Low-Carbohydrate and Low-Fat Diets on Weight Loss and Body Composition in Overweight Men and Women." *Nutr Metab* (Lond) 1(1) (2004): 13; PubMed PMID:15533250; PubMed Central PMCID: PMC538279.

39. Samaha, FF, N Iqbal, P Seshadri, KL Chicano, DA Daily, J McGrory, T Williams, M Williams, EJ Gracely, and L Stern. "A Low-Carbohydrate as Compared with a Low-Fat Diet in Severe Obesity." *N Engl J Med* 348(21) (2003): 2074–81; PubMed PMID: 12761364.

40. Greene, P, W Willett, et al. "Pilot 12-Week Feeding Weight Loss Comparison: Low-Fat vs. Low-Carbohydrate (Ketogenic) Diets" (abstract). *Obes Res* 11 (2003): A23.

41. Sondike, S., et al. "The Ketogenic Diet Increases Weight Loss but Not Cardiovascular Risk: A Randomized Controlled Trial." *Journal of Adolescent Health* 26 (2000): 91.

42. Levine, JA, NL Eberhardt, and MD Jensen. "Role of Nonexercise Activity Thermogenesis in Resistance to Fat Gain in Humans." *Science* 283(5399) (1999): 212–14; PubMed PMID: 9880251.

43. Lyon, DM, and DM Dunlop. "The Treatment of Obesity: A Comparison of the Effects of Diet and of Thyroid Extract." *QJM* 1 (1932): 331–52.

44. Dulloo, AG, CA Geissler, T Horton, A Collins, and DS Miller. "Normal Caffeine Consumption: Influence on Thermogenesis and Daily Energy Expenditure in Lean and Postobese Human Volunteers." *Am J Clin Nutr* 49(1) (1989): 44–50; PubMed PMID:2912010.

45. "Chapter 3: Weight Management." Health.gov, Your Portal to Health Information from the U.S. Government, http://www.health.gov/DietaryGuide lines/dga2005/document/html/chapter3.htm (accessed June 11, 2010).

46. *American Heart Association Complete Guide to Women's Heart Health: The Go Red for Women Way to Well-Being & Vitality*. New York: Clarkson Potter, 2009.

47. Haskell, WL, IM Lee, RR Pate, KE Powell, SN Blair, BA Franklin, CA Macera, GW Heath, PD Thompson, and A Bauman; American College of Sports Medicine; American Heart Association. "Physical Activity and Public Health: Updated Recommendation for Adults from the American College of Sports Medicine and the American Heart Association." *Circulation* 116(9) (2007): 1081–93; Epub August 1, 2007; PubMed PMID: 17671237.

48. McCullough, ML, D Feskanich, EB Rimm, EL Giovannucci, A Ascherio, JN Variyam, D Spiegelman, MJ Stampfer, and WC Willett. "Adherence to the Dietary Guidelines for Americans and Risk of Major Chronic Disease in Men." *Am J Clin Nutr* 72(5) (2000): 1223–31; PubMed PMID: 11063453.

49. Rony, Hugo R. *Obesity and Leanness* (London: Lea and Febiger, 1940).

50. Friedman, JM. "Modern Science versus the Stigma of Obesity." *Nat Med* 10(6) (2004): 563–69; review; PubMed PMID: 15170194.

51. Church, TS, CK Martin, AM Thompson, CP Earnest, CR Mikus, and SN Blair. "Changes in Weight, Waist Circumference, and Compensatory Responses with Different Doses of Exercise among Sedentary, Overweight Postmenopausal Women." *PLoS One* 4(2) (2009): e4515; Epub February 18, 2009; PubMed PMID: 19223984; PubMed Central PMCID: PMC2639700.

52. Caulfield, Timothy A. *The Cure for Everything: Untangling Twisted Messages about Health, Fitness, and Happiness*. Boston: Beacon Press, 2012.

53. National Soft Drink Association. "Soft Drinks: Balance, Variety, Moderation." http://www.nsda.org/softdrinks/CSDHealth/1layout.pdf.

54. Dwyer-Lindgren, L, G Freedman, RE Engell, TD Fleming, SS Lim, CJ Murray, and AH Mokdad. "Prevalence of Physical Activity and Obesity in US Counties, 2001–2011: A Road Map for Action." *Popul Health Metr* 11(1) (2013): 7; Epub ahead of print; PubMed PMID: 23842197. See also Institute for Health Metrics and Evaluation (IHME). "Obesity Continues to Rise in Nearly All Counties but Americans Becoming More Physically Active, Too," http://www.healthmetricsandevaluation.org/news-events/news -release/obesity-continues-rise-nearly-all-counties-americans-becoming (accessed July 10, 2013).

55. Whitehead, Saffron A., and Stephen Nussey. *Endocrinology: An Integrated Approach*. Oxford: BIOS, 2001, 122.

56. Petersen, L, P Schnohr, and TI Sørensen. "Longitudinal Study of the Long-Term Relation between Physical Activity and Obesity in Adults." *Int J Obes Relat Metab Disord* 28(1) (2004):105–12; PubMed PMID: 14647181.

57. Metcalf, BS, J Hosking, AN Jeffery, LD Voss, W Henley, and TJ Wilkin. "Fatness Leads to Inactivity, but Inactivity Does Not Lead to Fatness: A Longitudinal Study in Children" (EarlyBird 45). *Arch Dis Child* 96(10) (2011): 942–47; doi: 10.1136/adc.2009.175927; Epub June 23, 2010; PubMed PMID: 20573741.

58. Entin, Pauline. "History of Exercise Science." Northern Arizona University, http://www2.nau.edu, http://jan.ucc.nau.edu/pe/exs190web/exs190history .htm (accessed February 10, 2011).

59. Oliver, J. Eric. *Fat Politics: The Real Story behind America's Obesity Epidemic*. New ed. New York: Oxford University Press, 2006.

60. Nestle, M, and MF Jacobson. "Halting the Obesity Epidemic: A Public Health Policy Approach." *Public Health Rep* 115(1) (2000): 12–24; PubMed PMID: 10968581; PubMed Central PMCID: PMC1308552.

61. Roberts, Seth. *The Shangri-La Diet: The No Hunger Eat Anything Weight-Loss Plan*. Chicago: Perigee Trade, 2007.

62. Pontzer, H, DA Raichlen, BM Wood, AZ Mabulla, SB Racette, and FW Marlowe. "Hunter-Gatherer Energetics and Human Obesity." *PLoS One* 7(7) (2012): e40503; doi: 10.1371/journal.pone.0040503; Epub July 25, 2012; PubMed PMID: 22848382; PubMed Central PMCID: PMC3405064.

63. Feinman, RD, and EJ Fine. "'A Calorie Is a Calorie' Violates the Second Law of Thermodynamics." *Nutr J* 3 (2004 Jul 28): 9.

64. Krieger, JW, HS Sitren, MJ Daniels, and B Langkamp-Henken. "Effects of Variation in Protein and Carbohydrate Intake on Body Mass and Composition during Energy Restriction: A Meta-regression 1." *Am J Clin Nutr* 83(2) (2006): 260–74; PubMed PMID: 16469983.

65. Young, CM, SS Scanlan, HS Im, and L Lutwak. "Effect of Body Composition and Other Parameters in Obese Young Men of Carbohydrate Level of Reduction Diet." *Am J Clin Nutr* 24(3) (1971): 290–96; PubMed PMID: 5548734.

66. Benoit, FL, RL Martin, and RH Watten. "Changes in Body Composition during Weight Reduction in Obesity: Balance Studies Comparing Effects of Fasting and a Ketogenic Diet." *Ann Intern Med* 63(4) (1965): 604–12; PubMed PMID: 5838326.

67. Fine EJ, Feinman RD. "Thermodynamics of Weight Loss Diets." *Nutr Metab* (Lond) 1(1) (2004 Dec 8): 15;. PubMed PMID: 15588283; PubMed Central PMCID: PMC543577.

68. Boden, G, K Sargrad, C Homko, M Mozzoli, and TP Stein. "Effect of a

Low-Carbohydrate Diet on Appetite, Blood Glucose Levels, and Insulin Resistance in Obese Patients with Type 2 Diabetes." *Ann Intern Med* 142(6) (2005): 403–11; PubMed PMID: 15767618.

69. Weigle, DS, PA Breen, CC Matthys, HS Callahan, KE Meeuws, VR Burden, and JQ Purnell. "A High-Protein Diet Induces Sustained Reductions in Appetite, Ad Libitum Caloric Intake, and Body Weight Despite Compensatory Changes in Diurnal Plasma Leptin and Ghrelin Concentrations." *Am J Clin Nutr* 82(1) (2005): 41–48; PubMed PMID: 16002798.

70. Booth, DA, A Chase, and AT Campbell. "Relative Effectiveness of Protein in the Late Stages of Appetite Suppression in Man." *Physiol Behav* 5(11) (1970): 1299–1302; PubMed PMID: 5524514.

71. Hill, AJ, and JE Blundell. "Macronutrients and Satiety: The Effects of a High Protein or High Carbohydrate Meal on Subjective Motivation to Eat and Food Preferences." *Nutr Behav* 3 (1986): 133–44.

72. Barkeling, B, S Rössner, and H Björvell. "Effects of a High-Protein Meal (Meat) and a High-Carbohydrate Meal (Vegetarian) on Satiety Measured by Automated Computerized Monitoring of Subsequent Food Intake, Motivation to Eat and Food Preferences." *Int J Obes* 14(9) (1990): 743–51; PubMed PMID: 2228407.

73. Volek, Jeff, and Stephen D. Phinney. *The Art and Science of Low Carbohydrate Living: An Expert Guide to Making the Life-Saving Benefits of Carbohydrate Restriction Sustainable and Enjoyable.* Lexington, KY: Beyond Obesity, 2011.

74. Wertheimer, E, and B Shapiro. "The Physiology of Adipose Tissue." *Physiol Rev* 28 (1948): 451.

75. Brownell, Kelly, and Katherine Battle Horgen. *Food Fight.* 1st ed. New York: McGraw-Hill, 2004.

76. A sampling of supporting research includes the following studies: Harris, RB, and RJ Martin, "Specific Depletion of Body Fat in Parabiotic Partners of Tube-Fed Obese Rats," *Am J Physiol* 247(2 pt. 2) (1984): R380–86, PubMed PMID: 6431831; Harris, RB, and RJ Martin, "Influence of Diet on the Production of a 'Lipid-Depleting' Factor in Obese Parabiotic Rats," *J Nutr* 116(10) (1986): 2013–27, PubMed PMID: 3772528; Harris, RB, and RJ Martin, "Metabolic Response to a Specific Lipid-Depleting Factor in Parabiotic Rats," *Am J Physiol* 250(2 pt. 2) (1986): R276–86, PubMed PMID: 3511738; Havel, PJ, "Update on Adipocyte Hormones: Regulation of Energy Balance and Carbohydrate/Lipid Metabolism," *Diabetes* 53 suppl. 1 (2004): S143–51, review, PubMed PMID: 14749280; and Parameswaran, SV, AB Steffens, GR Hervey, and L de Ruiter, "Involvement of a Humoral Factor in Regulation of Body Weight in Parabiotic Rats," *Am J Physiol* 232(5) (1977): R150–57, PubMed PMID: 324294.

77. Kraemer, FB, and WJ Shen. "Hormone-Sensitive Lipase Knockouts." *Nutr Metab* (Lond) 3 (2006 Feb 10): 12; PubMed PMID: 16472389; PubMed Central PMCID: PMC1391915.

78. Polak, P, N Cybulski, JN Feige, J Auwerx, MA Rüegg, and MN Hall. "Adipose-Specific Knockout of Raptor Results in Lean Mice with Enhanced Mitochondrial Respiration." *Cell Metab* 8(5) (2008): 399–410; PubMed PMID: 19046571.

79. Havel, PJ. "Update on Adipocyte Hormones: Regulation of Energy Balance and Carbohydrate/Lipid Metabolism." *Diabetes* 53 suppl 1 (2004): S143–51; review; PubMed PMID: 14749280.

80. Le Magnen, J. "Is Regulation of Body Weight Elucidated." *Neurosci Biobehav Rev* 8(4) (1984): 515–22; review; PubMed PMID: 6392951.

81. Havel, PJ. "Dietary Fructose: Implications for Dysregulation of Energy Homeostasis and Lipid/Carbohydrate Metabolism." *Nutr Rev* 63(5) (2005): 133–57; review; PubMed PMID: 15971409.

82. Bruch, Hilde. *The Importance of Overweight*. New York: Norton, 1957.

83. Friedman, JM. "Modern Science versus the Stigma of Obesity." *Nat Med* 10(6) (2004): 563–69; review; PubMed PMID: 15170194.

84. Dabelea, D. "The Predisposition to Obesity and Diabetes in Offspring of Diabetic Mothers." *Diabetes Care* 30 suppl 2 (2007): S169–74; review; erratum in *Diabetes Care* 30(12) (2007): 3154; PubMed PMID: 17596467. The one-in-three statistic is from http://www.heart.org/HEARTORG/Getting Healthy/Overweight-in-Children_UCM_304054_Article.jsp and http://www .heart.org/idc/groups/heart-public/@wcm/@fc/documents/downloadable/ ucm_304175.pdf.

85. Eaton, SB, SB Eaton 3rd, and MJ Konner. "Paleolithic Nutrition Revisited: A Twelve-Year Retrospective on Its Nature and Implications." *Eur J Clin Nutr* 51(4) (1997): 207–16; review; PubMed PMID: 9104571.

86. Cordain L, SB Eaton, A Sebastian, N Mann, S Lindeberg, BA Watkins, JH O'Keefe, and J Brand-Miller. "Origins and Evolution of the Western Diet: Health Implications for the 21st Century." *Am J Clin Nutr* 81(2) (2005): 341–54; review; PubMed PMID: 15699220.

87. Boyd, S, Melvin Konner, Marjorie Shostak, and MD Eaton. *The Paleolithic Prescription: A Program of Diet and Exercise and a Design for Living*. New York: HarperCollins, 1989.

88. Skerrett, PJ, and WC Willett. *Eat, Drink, and Be Healthy: The Harvard Medical School Guide to Healthy Eating*. New York: Free Press, 2005.

89. Weinberg, SL. "The Diet-Heart Hypothesis: A Critique." *J Am Coll Cardiol* 43(5) (2004): 731–33; review; PubMed PMID: 14998608.

90. Jacobson, Michael F. *Nutrition Scoreboard*. New York: Avon Books, 1975.

91. E-mail correspondence with Donald Layman, October 3, 2012.

92. Nestle, Marion. *Food Politics: How the Food Industry Influences Nutrition and Health*. Rev. and expanded ed. California Studies in Food and Culture. Berkeley: University of California Press, 2002.

93. Skerrett and Willett. *Eat, Drink, and Be Healthy*.

94. Ottoboni, A, and F Ottoboni. "The Food Guide Pyramid: Will the Defects Be Corrected?" *J Am Phys Surg* 9 (2004): 109–13.

95. Truswell, AS. "Evolution of Dietary Recommendations, Goals, and Guidelines." *Am J Clin Nutr* 45(5 suppl) (1987): 1060–72; review; PubMed PMID: 3554965.

96. Harper, AE. "Dietary Goals—A Skeptical View." *Am J Clin Nutr* 31(2) (1978): 310–21; review; PubMed PMID: 341685.

97. Truswell. "Evolution of Dietary Recommendations."

98. Council for Responsible Nutrition. "Resolution Endorsing Dietary Goals for the United States Presented to Members of the Senate Select Committee on Nutrition and Human Needs." May 12, 1977. *Comm Nutr Inst Weekly Report* 7, no. 21 (1977): 4.

99. Yerushalmy, J, and HE Hilleboe. "Fat in the Diet and Mortality from Heart Disease: A Methodologic Note." *N Y State J Med* 57(14) (1957): 2343–54; PubMed PMID:13441073.

100. Enig, Mary G., and Sally Fallon. *Eat Fat, Lose Fat: The Healthy Alternative to Trans Fats*. New York: Plume, 2006.

101. Skerrett and Willett. *Eat, Drink, and Be Healthy*.

102. Siri-Tarino, PW, Q Sun, FB Hu, and RM Krauss. "Meta-Analysis of Prospective Cohort Studies Evaluating the Association of Saturated Fat with Cardiovascular Disease." *Am J Clin Nutr* (2010); Epub ahead of print, January 13, 2010; PubMed PMID: 20071648.

103. Multiple Risk Factor Intervention Trial Research Group. "Multiple Risk Factor Intervention Trial: Risk Factor Changes and Mortality Results." *JAMA* 248(12) (1982): 1465–77; PubMed PMID: 7050440.

104. Howard, BV, L Van Horn, J Hsia, JE Manson, ML Stefanick, S Wassertheil-Smoller, LH Kuller, AZ LaCroix, RD Langer, NL Lasser, CE Lewis, MC Limacher, KL Margolis, WJ Mysiw, JK Ockene, LM Parker, MG Perri, L Phillips, RL Prentice, J Robbins, JE Rossouw, GE Sarto, IJ Schatz, LG Snetselaar, VJ Stevens, LF Tinker, M Trevisan, MZ Vitolins, GL Anderson, AR Assaf, T Bassford, SA Beresford, HR Black, RL Brunner, RG Brzyski, B Caan, RT Chlebowski, M Gass, I Granek, P Greenland, J Hays, D Heber, G Heiss, SL Hendrix, FA Hubbell, KC Johnson, and JM Kotchen. "Low-Fat Dietary Pattern and Risk of Cardiovascular Disease: The Women's Health Initiative Randomized Controlled Dietary Modification Trial." *JAMA* 295(6) (2006): 655–66; PubMed PMID: 16467234.

105. Willett, W. "Challenges for Public Health Nutrition in the 1990s." *Am J*

Public Health 80(11) (1990): 1295–98; PubMed PMID: 2240291; PubMed Central PMCID: PMC1404889.

106. Hu, FB, JE Manson, and WC Willett. "Types of Dietary Fat and Risk of Coronary Heart Disease: A Critical Review." *J Am Coll Nutr* 20(1) (2001): 5–19; review.

107. Taubes, Gary. *Good Calories, Bad Calories: Challenging the Conventional Wisdom on Diet, Weight Control, and Disease*. New York: Alfred A. Knopf, 2007.

108. Skerrett, PJ, and WC Willett. *Eat, Drink, and Be Healthy: The Harvard Medical School Guide to Healthy Eating*. New York: Free Press, 2005.

109. Ravnskov, Uffe. *Fat and Cholesterol Are Good for You*. N.p.: GP, 2009.

110. Centers for Disease Control and Prevention (CDC). "Trends in Intake of Energy and Macronutrients—United States, 1971–2000." *MMWR Morb Mortal Wkly Rep* 53(4) (2004): 80–82; PubMed PMID: 14762332.

111. *Dietary Reference Intakes for Energy, Carbohydrate, Fiber, Fat, Fatty Acids, Cholesterol, Protein, and Amino Acids*. Washington, DC: National Academies Press, 2005.

112. Nestle, Marion. *Food Politics: How the Food Industry Influences Nutrition and Health*. Rev. and expanded ed. California Studies in Food and Culture. Berkeley: University of California Press, 2002.

113. Carey, Anne R., and Paul Trap. "Stretching the Truth." *USA Today*, January 13, 2011, USA Today Snapshots, 1.

114. St Jeor, ST, BV Howard, TE Prewitt, V Bovee, T Bazzarre, and RH Eckel; Nutrition Committee of the Council on Nutrition, Physical Activity, and Metabolism of the American Heart Association. "Dietary Protein and Weight Reduction: A Statement for Healthcare Professionals from the Nutrition Committee of the Council on Nutrition, Physical Activity, and Metabolism of the American Heart Association." *Circulation* 104(15) (2001): 1869–74; PubMed PMID: 11591629.

115. "Status of Articles Offered to the General Public for the Control or Reduction of Blood Cholesterol Levels and for the Prevention and Treatment of Heart and Artery Disease under the Federal Food, Drug, and Cosmetic Act." *Federal Register*, December 12, 1959.

116. Gordon, T, WP Castelli, MC Hjortland, WB Kannel, and TR Dawber. "High Density Lipoprotein as a Protective Factor against Coronary Heart Disease: The Framingham Study." *Am J Med* 62 (1977): 707–14.

117. Ravnskov, U. "Cholesterol Lowering Trials in Coronary Heart Disease: Frequency of Citation and Outcome." *BMJ* 305(6844) (1992 Jul 4): 15–19; erratum in *BMJ* 305(6852) (1992 Aug 29): 505; PubMed PMID: 1638188; PubMed Central PMCID: PMC1882525.

118. Sacks, FM, GA Bray, VJ Carey, SR Smith, DH Ryan, SD Anton, K McManus,

CM Champagne, LM Bishop, N Laranjo, MS Leboff, JC Rood, L de Jonge, FL Greenway, CM Loria, E Obarzanek, and DA Williamson. "Comparison of Weight-Loss Diets with Different Compositions of Fat, Protein, and Carbohydrates." *N Engl J Med* 360(9) (2009): 859–73; doi: 10.1056/NEJMoa080 4748; PubMed PMID: 19246357; PubMed Central PMCID: PMC2763382.

119. Castelli, WP, "Cholesterol and Lipids in the Risk of Coronary Artery Disease—The Framingham Heart Study." *Can J Cardiol* 4 (1988): 5A–10A; Gordon, T, WP Castelli, MC Hjortland, WB Kannel, and TR Dawber, "High-Density Lipoprotein as a Protective Factor against Coronary Heart Disease—The Framingham Study." *Am J Med* 62 (1977): 707–14; Gordon, DJ, JL Probstfield, RJ Garrison, et al., "High-Density Lipoprotein Cholesterol and Cardiovascular Disease—Four Prospective American Studies." *Circulation* 79 (1989): 8–15; Sharrett, AR, CM Ballantyne, SA Coady, et al., "Coronary Heart Disease Prediction from Lipoprotein Cholesterol Levels, Triglycerides, Lipoprotein(a), Apolipoproteins A-I and B, and HDL Density Subfractions—The Atherosclerosis Risk in Communities (ARIC) Study." *Circulation* 104 (2001): 1108–13.

120. Mozaffarian, D, and DS Ludwig. "Dietary Guidelines in the 21st Century—a Time for Food." *JAMA* 304(6) (2010): 681–82; doi: 10.1001/jama.2010. 1116; PubMed PMID: 20699461.

121. http://www.gmabrands.com/publicpolicy/docs/Correspondence.cfm?Doc ID=1123&.

122. *Soft Drinks and Nutrition*. Washington, DC: National Soft Drink Association, n.d.

123. "The National Institutes of Health: Public Servant or Private Marketer?" *Los Angeles Times*, http://articles.latimes.com/2004/dec/22/nation/na-nih22 (accessed April 28, 2010).

124. Popkin, Barry. *The World Is Fat: The Fads, Trends, Policies, and Products That Are Fattening the Human Race*. New York: Avery, 2008.

125. Guyenet, Stephan. "Whole Health Source: By 2606, the US Diet Will Be 100 Percent Sugar." *Whole Health Source*. http://wholehealthsource .blogspot.com/2012/02/by-2606-us-diet-will-be-100-percent.html (accessed February 19, 2012).

126. Avena, NM, P Rada, and BG Hoebel. "Evidence for Sugar Addiction: Behavioral and Neurochemical Effects of Intermittent, Excessive Sugar Intake." *Neurosci Biobehav Rev* 32(1) (2008): 20–39; Epub May 18, 2007; review; PubMed PMID: 17617461; PubMed Central PMCID: PMC2235907.

127. Colantuoni, C, P Rada, J McCarthy, C Patten, NM Avena, A Chadeayne, and BG Hoebel. "Evidence That Intermittent, Excessive Sugar Intake Causes Endogenous Opioid Dependence." *Obes Res* 10(6) (2002): 478–88; PubMed PMID: 12055324.

128. Avena et al. "Evidence for Sugar Addiction."

129. Hoebel, BG, NM Avena, ME Bocarsly, and P Rada. "Natural Addiction: A Behavioral and Circuit Model Based on Sugar Addiction in Rats." *J Addict Med* 3(1) (2009): 33–41; doi: 10.1097/ADM.0b013e31819aa621; PubMed PMID: 21768998.

130. "Tobacco CEO's Statement to Congress." UCSF Academic Senate. http://senate.ucsf.edu/tobacco/executives1994congress.html (accessed July 18, 2010).

131. National Soft Drink Association website. Available at http://www.nsda.org/softdrinks/CSDHealth/Index.html.

132. "Daily Doc: Lorillard, Aug 30, 1978: 'The Base of Our Business Is the High School Student.'" Tobacco.org: Welcome, http://www.tobacco.org/Documents/dd/ddbasebusiness.html (accessed July 18, 2010).

133. Horovitz, B. "McDonald's Rediscovers Its Future with Kids." *USA Today*, April 18, 1997.

134. "Jan. 4, 1954: TIRC Announced." Tobacco.org: Welcome, http://www.tobacco.org/History/540104frank.html (accessed July 18, 2010).

135 Hays, CL, and DG McNeil Jr. "Putting Africa on Coke's Map." *New York Times*, May 26, 1998, D1.

136. "Jan. 4, 1954: TIRC Announced," http://archive.tobacco.org/History/54010frank.html.

137. National Soft Drink Association website.

138. Brownell, Kelly, and Katherine Battle Horgen. *Food Fight*. 1st ed. New York: McGraw-Hill, 2004.

139. Yudkin, John. *Sweet and Dangerous*. Washington DC: National Health Federation, 1978.

140. Boyd, S, Melvin Konner, Marjorie Shostak, and MD Eaton. *The Paleolithic Prescription: A Program of Diet and Exercise and a Design for Living*. New York: HarperCollins, 1989.

141. McGuff, Doug. "Body by Science—Especially for Women." Body by Science, http://www.bodybyscience.net/home.html/?page_id=301 (accessed February 12, 2012).

142. Klein, S, NF Sheard, X Pi-Sunyer, A Daly, J Wylie-Rosett, K Kulkarni, NG Clark; American Diabetes Association; North American Association for the Study of Obesity; American Society for Clinical Nutrition. "Weight Management through Lifestyle Modification for the Prevention and Management of Type 2 Diabetes: Rationale and Strategies: A Statement of the American Diabetes Association, the North American Association for the Study of Obesity, and the American Society for Clinical Nutrition." *Diabetes Care* 27(8) (2004): 2067–73; review; PubMed PMID:15277443.

143. Shai, I, D Schwarzfuchs, Y Henkin, DR Shahar, S Witkow, I Greenberg,

R Golan, D Fraser, A Bolotin, H Vardi, O Tangi-Rozental, R Zuk-Ramot, B Sarusi, D Brickner, Z Schwartz, E Sheiner, R Marko, E Katorza, J Thiery, GM Fiedler, M Blüher, M Stumvoll, and MJ Stampfer; Dietary Intervention Randomized Controlled Trial (DIRECT) Group. "Weight Loss with a Low-Carbohydrate, Mediterranean, or Low-Fat Diet." *N Engl J Med* 359(3) (2008): 229–41; erratum in: *N Engl J Med* 361(27) (2009): 2681; PubMed PMID: 18635428.

144. *Dietary Reference Intakes for Energy, Carbohydrate, Fiber, Fat, Fatty Acids, Cholesterol, Protein, and Amino Acids.* Washington, DC: National Academies Press, 2005.

145. Layman, DK, P Clifton, MC Gannon, RM Krauss, and FQ Nuttall. "Protein in Optimal Health: Heart Disease and Type 2 Diabetes." *Am J Clin Nutr* 87(5) (2008): 1571S–75S; review; PubMed PMID: 18469290.

146. Eaton, SB, SB Eaton 3rd, and MJ Konner. "Paleolithic Nutrition Revisited: A Twelve-Year Retrospective on Its Nature and Implications." *Eur J Clin Nutr* 51(4) (1997): 207–16; review; PubMed PMID: 9104571.

147. Skerrett, PJ, and WC Willett. *Eat, Drink, and Be Healthy: The Harvard Medical School Guide to Healthy Eating.* New York: Free Press, 2005.

148. Campbell, T. Colin, and Thomas M. Campbell. *The China Study: The Most Comprehensive Study of Nutrition Ever Conducted and the Startling Implications for Diet, Weight Loss, and Long-Term Health.* Dallas, Tex.: BenBella Books, 2005.

149. Jaminet, Paul, and Shou Jaminet. *Perfect Health Diet: Regain Health and Lose Weight by Eating the Way You Were Meant to Eat.* New York: Scribner, 2012.

150. Hu, FB, and WC Willard. "Reply to TC Campbell." *Am J Clin Nutr* 71 (2000): 850–51 (letter).

151. Wang, Y, MA Crawford, J Chen, J Li, K Ghebremeskel, TC Campbell, W Fan, R Parker, and J Leyton. "Fish Consumption, Blood Docosahexaenoic Acid and Chronic Diseases in Chinese Rural Populations." *Comp Biochem Physiol A Mol Integr Physiol* 136(1) (2003): 127–40; review; PubMed PMID: 14527635.

152. Fuhrman, Joel. "What You Need to Know about Vegetarian or Vegan Diets." DrFuhrman.com, http://www.drfuhrman.com/library/article5.aspx (accessed May 12, 2012).

153. Hu, FB, and WC Willett. "Optimal Diets for Prevention of Coronary Heart Disease." *JAMA* 288(20) (2002): 2569–78; review; PubMed PMID: 12444864.

154. Masterjohn, Chris. "The Curious Case of Campbell's Rats—Does Protein Deficiency Prevent Cancer?" The Weston A. Price Foundation, http://www.westonaprice.org/blogs/2010/09/22/the-curious-case-of-campbells-rats-does-protein-deficiency-prevent-cancer (accessed December 17, 2011).

155. Westerterp-Plantenga, MS, A Nieuwenhuizen, D Tomé, S Soenen, and

KR Westerterp. "Dietary Protein, Weight Loss, and Weight Maintenance." *Annu Rev Nutr* 29 (2009): 21–41; review; PubMed PMID: 19400750.

156. Hu, FB, JE Manson, and WC Willett. "Types of Dietary Fat and Risk of Coronary Heart Disease: A Critical Review." *J Am Coll Nutr* 20(1) (2001): 5–19; review; PubMed PMID: 11293467.

157. Melov, S, MA Tarnopolsky, K Beckman, K Felkey, and A Hubbard. "Resistance Exercise Reverses Aging in Human Skeletal Muscle." *PLoS One* 2(5) (2007): e465; PubMed PMID: 17520024; PubMed Central PMCID: PMC1866181.

158. McGuff, Doug, and John R. Little. *Body by Science: A Research Based Program to Get the Results You Want in 12 Minutes a Week.* New York: McGraw-Hill, 2009.

159. Caulfield, Timothy A. *The Cure for Everything: Untangling Twisted Messages about Health, Fitness, and Happiness.* Boston: Beacon Press, 2012.

160. Kolata, Gina Bari. *Ultimate Fitness: The Quest for Truth about Exercise and Health.* New York: Farrar, Straus and Giroux, 2003.

161. Izumiya, Y, T Hopkins, C Morris, K Sato, L Zeng, J Viereck, JA Hamilton, N Ouchi, NK LeBrasseur, and K Walsh. "Fast/Glycolytic Muscle Fiber Growth Reduces Fat Mass and Improves Metabolic Parameters in Obese Mice." *Cell Metab* 7(2) (2008): 159–72; PubMed PMID: 18249175.

162. Oliver, J. Eric. *Fat Politics: The Real Story behind America's Obesity Epidemic.* New ed. New York: Oxford University Press, 2006.

163. Kolata, Gina Bari. *Ultimate Fitness: The Quest for Truth about Exercise and Health.* New York: Farrar, Straus and Giroux, 2003.

164. Izumiya, Y, T Hopkins, C Morris, K Sato, L Zeng, J Viereck, JA Hamilton, N Ouchi, NK LeBrasseur, and K Walsh. "Fast/Glycolytic Muscle Fiber Growth Reduces Fat Mass and Improves Metabolic Parameters in Obese Mice." *Cell Metab* 7(2) (2008): 159–72; PubMed PMID: 18249175.

165. Carpinelli, RN, and RM Otto. "Strength Training: Single versus Multiple Sets." *Sports Med* 26(2) (1998): 73–84; review; PubMed PMID: 9777681.

166. Roig, M, K O'Brien, G Kirk, R Murray, P McKinnon, B Shadgan, and WD Reid. "The Effects of Eccentric versus Concentric Resistance Training on Muscle Strength and Mass in Healthy Adults: A Systematic Review with Meta-Analysis." *Br J Sports Med* 43(8) (2009): 556–68; doi: 10.1136/bjsm.2008.051417; Epub November 3, 2008; review; PubMed PMID: 18981046.

167. Reeves, ND, CN Maganaris, S Longo, and MV Narici. "Differential Adaptations to Eccentric versus Conventional Resistance Training in Older Humans." *Exp Physiol* 94(7) (2009): 825–33; Epub April 24, 2009; PubMed PMID: 19395657.

168. Babraj, JA, NB Vollaard, C Keast, FM Guppy, G Cottrell, and JA Timmons.

"Extremely Short Duration High Intensity Interval Training Substantially Improves Insulin Action in Young Healthy Males." *BMC Endocr Disord* 9 (2009 Jan 28): 3; PubMed PMID: 19175906; PubMed Central PMCID: PMC2640399.

169. Earnest, CP. "Exercise Interval Training: An Improved Stimulus for Improving the Physiology of Pre-Diabetes." *Med Hypotheses* 71(5) (2008): 752–61; Epub August 15, 2008; PubMed PMID: 18707813.

170. Irving, BA, CK Davis, DW Brock, JY Weltman, D Swift, EJ Barrett, GA Gaesser, and A Weltman. "Effect of Exercise Training Intensity on Abdominal Visceral Fat and Body Composition." *Med Sci Sports Exerc* 40(11) (2008): 1863–72; PubMed PMID:18845966; PubMed Central PMCID: PMC2730190.

171. McGuff, Doug, and John R. Little. *Body by Science: A Research Based Program to Get the Results You Want in 12 Minutes a Week*. New York: McGraw-Hill, 2009.

172. Sesso, HD, RS Paffenbarger Jr, and IM Lee. "Physical Activity and Coronary Heart Disease in Men: The Harvard Alumni Health Study." *Circulation* 102(9) (2000): 975–80; PubMed PMID: 10961960.

173. Paffenbarger, RS, Jr, and IM Lee. "Intensity of Physical Activity Related to Incidence of Hypertension and All-Cause Mortality: An Epidemiological View." *Blood Press Monit* 2(3) (1997): 115–23; PubMed PMID: 10234104.

174. Lee, IM, HD Sesso, Y Oguma, and RS Paffenbarger Jr. "Relative Intensity of Physical Activity and Risk of Coronary Heart Disease." *Circulation* 107(8) (2003): 1110–16; PubMed PMID: 12615787.

175. Haskell, WL, IM Lee, RR Pate, KE Powell, SN Blair, BA Franklin, CA Macera, GW Heath, PD Thompson, and A Bauman; American College of Sports Medicine; American Heart Association. "Physical Activity and Public Health: Updated Recommendation for Adults from the American College of Sports Medicine and the American Heart Association." *Circulation* 116(9) (2007): 1081–93; Epub August 1, 2007; PubMed PMID: 17671237.

176. Haram, PM, OJ Kemi, SJ Lee, MØ Bendheim, QY al-Share, HL Waldum, LJ Gilligan, LG Koch, SL Britton, SM Najjar, and U Wisløff. "Aerobic Interval Training vs. Continuous Moderate Exercise in the Metabolic Syndrome of Rats Artificially Selected for Low Aerobic Capacity." *Cardiovasc Res* 81(4) (2009): 723–32; Epub December 1, 2008; PubMed PMID: 19047339; PubMed Central PMCID: PMC2642601.

177. Coyle, EF. "Very Intense Exercise-Training Is Extremely Potent and Time Efficient: A Reminder." *J Appl Physiol* 98(6) (2005): 1983–84; PubMed PMID:15894535.

178. Branden, Nathaniel. *The Six Pillars of Self-Esteem*. New York: Bantam, 1994.

179. Yudkin, John. *Sweet and Dangerous*. Washington DC: National Health Federation, 1978.

180. American Heart Association. "Understanding Childhood Obesity." www.heart .org/HEARTORG/GettingHealthy/Overweight-in-Children_UCM_304054 _Article.jsp.

181. Carpinelli, RN. "Berger in Retrospect: Effect of Varied Strength Training Programmes on Strength." *Br J Sports Med* 36(5) (2002): 319–24; review; PubMed PMID: 12351327; PubMed Central PMCID: PMC1724552.

182. Babraj, JA, NB Vollaard, C Keast, FM Guppy, G Cottrell, and JA Timmons. "Extremely Short Duration High Intensity Interval Training Substantially Improves Insulin Action in Young Healthy Males." *BMC Endocr Disord* 9 (2009 Jan 28): 3; PubMed PMID: 19175906; PubMed Central PMCID: PMC2640399.

183. Ravnskov, Uffe, and Joel M. Kauffman. *Fat and Cholesterol Are Good for You*. N.p.: GP, 2009.

Index

Page numbers of illustrations, charts, and graphs appear in italics.